PF625299

Library of
Davidson College

On the Development of Developmental Psychology

Contributions to
Human Development

Vol. 8

Series Editor
John A. Meacham, Buffalo, N.Y.

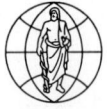

S. Karger · Basel · München · Paris · London · New York · Sydney

On the Development of Developmental Psychology

Volume Editors
Deanna Kuhn, New York, N.Y., and
John A. Meacham, Buffalo, N.Y.

1 figure, 1983

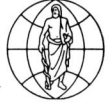

S. Karger · Basel · München · Paris · London · New York · Sydney

Contributions to Human Development

Vol. 6: The Play of Children: Current Theory and Research
Pepler, D.J., Mississauga, and Rubin, K.H., Waterloo (eds.)
X + 158 p., 1 fig., 11 tab., 1982. ISBN 3-8055-3540-6
Vol. 7: Henry, R.M., Wollongong
The Psychodynamic Foundations of Morality
ISBN 3-8055-3603-8

National Library of Medicine, Cataloging in Publication
 On the development of developmental psychology/
 volume editors, Deanna Kuhn and John A. Meacham. – Basel; New York: Karger, 1983.
 (Contributions to human development; v. 8)
 1. Human Development I. Kuhn, Deanna II. Meacham, J.A. III. Series
 W1 C0778S v. 8 [BF 713 058]
 ISBN 3-8055-3568-6

All rights reserved
 No part of this publication may be translated into other languages, reproduced or utilized in any form or by any means, electronic or mechanical, including photocopying, recording, microcopying, or by any information storage and retrieval system, without permission in writing from the publisher.

© Copyright 1983 by S. Karger AG, P.O. Box, CH-4009 Basel (Switzerland)
 Printed in Switzerland by gdz Genossenschaftsdruckerei Zürich
 ISBN 3-8055-3568-6

Contents

Preface VII

Kitchener, R.F. (Fort Collins, Colo.): Changing Conceptions of the Philosophy of Science and the Foundations of Developmental Psychology 1
Youniss, J. (Washington, D.C.): Beyond Ideology to the Universals of Development 31
Siegel, A.W. (Houston, Tex.); *Bisanz, J.; Bisanz, G.L.* (Edmonton): Developmental Analysis: A Strategy for the Study of Psychological Change 53
Kuhn, D. (Cambridge, Mass.): On the Dual Executive and Its Significance in the Development of Developmental Psychology   81
Meacham, J.A. (Buffalo, N.Y.): Wisdom and the Context of Knowledge: Knowing that One Doesn't Know 111
Newman, D.; Riel, M.; Martin, L.M.W. (La Jolla, Calif.): Cultural Practices and Piagetian Theory: The Impact of a Cross-Cultural Research Program 135

Author Index 155
Subject Index 158

Preface

The present volume, despite its title, does not provide a history of developmental psychology. In recent years, a number of histories of developmental psychology have appeared, for example by *Sears* [1975] and *Senn* [1975] in the area of child development and by *Charles* [1970] and *Reinert* [1979] in the area of adult development and aging. For the most part, however, these histories concern the earlier stages in the development of the discipline. The present volume, in contrast, focuses on the recent past, the present, and the projected future of developmental psychology. The guiding premise is that developmental psychologists should demand of themselves an increased reflectivity on what it is that they are doing, both individually and collectively as a discipline and, moreover, that this reflection must be undertaken from an historical frame of reference. Thus, each chapter includes as a primary theme reflections *about* developmental theory or method, in historical perspective, rather than merely contributions *to* one or the other.

The authors of this volume are, for the most part, developmental psychologists. Their chapters represent diverse viewpoints within developmental psychology and provide perspectives on current theoretical and methodological issues in the study of social, personality, and cognitive development from infancy through old age. Thus, this volume is most appropriate for advanced undergraduate students, graduate students, and academicians and researchers in developmental psychology, as well as in related areas of sociology and education. In addition, the volume may be of interest to historians, to those concerned with the sociology of science, as well as to scholars in any of the social or physical sciences who are seeking discussions of the historical development of disciplines and the implications of this development for contemporary theory and research.

It might be expected that developmental psychologists, whose efforts are directed towards understanding sequences of changes within individuals, would also turn their attention to sequences of development in their own activities as theorists and researchers. By and large, however, neither developmental psychology nor psychology overall has tended to engage in such reflection. Psychologists writing about themselves in the present tense is a relatively rare occurrence. Moreover, to the extent that such self-contemplation has occurred, psychologists by and large have not viewed themselves and their current activities within the context of the discipline's own history. Both theorists and researchers have tended to absorb themselves in the conceptual or empirical issues of current concern without a sufficient appreciation of the social and historical contexts in which their own attention to these issues is embedded. It may be more true than the contributors to this volume would like to believe that present-day students, teachers, and reseachers can safely ignore all but the past few years of theory and research and still prosper by prevailing standards.

On the positive side, there has come to be a greater appreciation of the fact that the sequence of development of individual persons is embedded within particular historical and social contexts [*Kessen,* 1979]. There is now considerable interest in what the sequence of individual development was like in earlier times and what factors caused it to be the way it was, as reflected, for example, in *Aries'* [1962] history of family life, *Gadlin's* [1978] review of child discipline in the 19th century, and *Kett's* [1977] study of the emergence of adolescence as a life stage. Yet few writers have focused on more recent times, although *Elder's* [1974] follow-up of children born during the great depression is a notable exception. The implication of these historical studies is that an understanding of development – including description and explanation – achieved during earlier periods will not necessarily be valid for later periods. Indeed, this point is now widely accepted.

Yet it is rare for developmentalists to make the logical extension and regard their own activities as scholars as equally embedded in social and historical contexts. To the extent such recognition exists, it tends to remain at the periphery of the discipline's activities and awareness, unintegrated with ongoing work. It was the belief of *Klaus Riegel* that we know about human development only through our own actions of constructing successive interpretations which provide meaning and, at the same time, come between ourselves and the objective facts. Thus, what is called for in psychology is the study of the sequence of these interpretations [*Riegel,* 1979]. At the very least, the discipline needs, and stands to benefit from, such reflectivity regarding its past and future development, a reflectivity that includes a sense of the dependence of our present theories and methods upon our own past and present social and historical circumstances. Ideally this reflectivity will become integrated and reciprocally coordinated with our ongoing work, rather than remaining at the periphery of it.

In addition, the intent of these chapters is to consider what influences have altered the course of theoretical and empirical work in developmental psychology: for example, new empirical findings, new research methods, critiques of existing theories or methods, social, political, and economic contexts, fertilization from other disciplines, the exhaustion of paradigms, falsification of theories, etc. This discussion is extended from the present to the future, and the authors consider what may be some historical turning points or alternative courses for contemporary developmental psychology. To accomplish these intentions necessitates an evaluation of the success of developmental theories relative to various functions or purposes of theories: integration, explanation, generation of new questions, etc. *Gergen* [1980] has suggested that developmental psychology is undergoing a change in its perception of the critical function of theory, from prediction and control to challenging prevailing views, suggesting alternative solutions to existing problems, elaborating alternative forms of social action, and sustaining cultural values.

A recurring theme in this set of commentaries on the progress of developmental psychology is that the positivist doctrine prevalent in the philosophy of science in the middle of the 20th century has not served the field of developmental psychology well as a model for its efforts. *Kitchener,* whose chapter focuses most centrally on this theme, illustrates the reflection within developmental psychology of numerous key tenets of 1950s positivism, e.g. that observation is theory-free and that all theoretical constructs must be linked to specific empirical operations. *Kitchener* accuses developmental psychologists of endorsing methodological behaviorism as a research paradigm, equating it even with 'scientific method'. He goes on to explain why the tenets of 1950s positivism have been rejected by the philosophy of science, making it all the more paradoxical that they continue to be adhered to as a model of scientific inquiry by developmental psychologists.

Youniss characterizes the limiting effects its adherence to positivism has had on developmental psychology. The positivist focus on methods of data collection and analysis, he claims, has led developmental psychologists to become chroniclers of the 'here-and-now'. What is gained in so doing is confidence in the verifiability of their observations. What is lost, *Youniss* argues, however, is generality of one's findings – they remain tied to a particular time and place. Also lost is the potential fertilization from intellectual traditions that offer insights that cannot be achieved from observation of here-and-now behavior.

In a more positive and prescriptive vein, both *Kitchener* and *Youniss,* as well as several of the other authors, emphasize that both theory and method evolve historically. What is called for, therefore, they argue, is conceptualization of both its subject matter and the discipline itself in a dynamic, developmental perspective. *Youniss* criticizes facile rejection of theories as soon as they have been recognized as having ties to a particular historical-cultural-ideological context. He argues, rather, for use of methods of sociological and historical analysis in understanding both the subject matter of developmental psychology and its own dynamic development. *Kitchener* points out that postpositivistic philosophy of science has itself become increasingly developmental, recognizing the importance of a reciprocal interaction between itself and several of the social sciences, particularly, *Kitchener* claims, developmental psychology.

The chapter by *Siegel, Bisanz, and Bisanz* is most specific in its prescriptions for developmental psychology. They argue that to be most fruitful, developmental psychology should more clearly define itself as a subdiscipline with shared goals and methods. To regard developmental psychology as simply the study of change is too broad and undifferentiating, they claim. Drawing on the writings of *Herbert Spencer,* they define a method of developmental analysis that they believe addresses the field's need for a conceptual framework emphasizing change, rather than static representations. Their intent is to suggest a framework for research and theory that can provide a common agenda for developmental psychologists in diverse areas.

The remaining three chapters focus their analyses on specific subdomains or research traditions within developmental psychology, in a way, nevertheless, that reflects on the field as a whole. *Kuhn* addresses the subfield of cognitive development as it has evolved over the past 25 years, reflecting on the rapid rise and then decline in the popularity of

Piaget's theory and the recent rise to prominence of information-processing models as an apparent 'replacement' for *Piaget*. Particular attention is given to the recent theoretical effort by *Case* [1978a, b] to integrate the best of the Piagetian and information-processing worlds, an effort which according to Kuhn's analysis reflects the long-standing tension between causal and intentional models of human action. *Kuhn* uses this analysis as an example to support her claim that we tend to take our themes too seriously in developmental psychology, allowing our enthusiasm for them to blind us to their limitations and boundaries and causing a narrowing of perspective on the problems we set out to address. The field would profit, she claims, from increased recognition that there exist some enduring questions in psychology.

Meacham analyzes the constructs of intelligence and knowledge as they have evolved both within the field of developmental psychology and more broadly. Like those of *Youniss* and *Kitchener*, *Meacham's* chapter draws parallels between the development of the individual and the development of scientific disciplines such as developmental psychology. Intelligence and knowledge are particularly important and revealing constructs to trace in any analysis of developmental psychology, *Meacham* states, especially to the extent that they may illuminate the discipline's own knowledge-seeking activities. *Meacham* points out the correspondence between conceptions of the individual and conceptions of intelligence across different cultures. He argues for a contextual, rather than accumulative, conception of knowledge development and proposes a model of knowledge development that reflects this conception.

The chapter by *Newman, Riel, and Martin* is devoted to an analysis of cross-cultural methodology as an extremely important testing ground for developmental theory. They describe the program of cross-cultural research prescribed by *Piaget* as a test of his theory and examine how this research program has fared in practice. *Newman* et al. come to the conclusion that it is inadequate to categorize cultures on some global, quantitative dimension of 'amount' of experience they provide, a practice that has arisen from interpretations of Piagetian theory. Cultures differ on a multitude of different dimensions, and a focus on the testing of Piagetian hypotheses has led away from an examination of these differences. *Newman* et al. call for more specific analysis of cultures and cultural practices, if the field of cross-cultural developmental research is to progress, and suggest the value of a Vygotskian framework in carrying out this task.

Although the chapters in this book are informed by the authors' interpretations of the history of developmental psychology, the emphasis is upon understanding changes in theory and method as these are occurring now; although the chapters provide some strong hints as to future advances in developmental psychology, the primary contribution is to raise questions regarding what changes are taking place currently, how these can be understood in an historical context, and what these changes might imply with respect to the continuing development of developmental psychology.

References

Aries, P.: Centuries of childhood: a social history of family life (Knopf, New York 1962).
Case, R.: Intellectual development from birth to adolescence: a neo-Piagetian interpretation; in Siegler, Children's thinking: What develops? (Erlbaum, Hillsdale 1978a).
Case, R.: Piaget and beyond: toward a developmentally based theory and technology of instruction; in Glaser, Advances in instructional psychology, vol. 1 (Erlbaum, Hillsdale 1978b).
Charles, D.C.: Historical antecedents of life-span developmental psychology; in Goulet, Baltes, Life-span developmental psychology: research and theory (Academic Press, New York 1970).
Elder, G.H., Jr.: Children of the great depression (University of Chicago Press, Chicago 1974).
Gadlin, H.: Child discipline and the pursuit of self; in Reese, Lipsitt, Advances in child development and behavior, vol. 13 (Academic Press, New York 1978).
Gergen, K.J.: The emerging crisis in life-span developmental theory; in Baltes, Brim, Life-span development and behavior, vol. 3 (Academic Press, New York 1980).
Kessen, W.: The American child and other cultural inventions. Am. Psychol. *34:* 815–820 (1979).
Kett, J.: Rites of passage (Basic Books, New York 1977).
Reinert, G.: Prolegomena to a history of life-span developmental psychology; in Baltes, Brim, Life-span development and behavior, vol. 2 (Academic Press, New York 1979).
Riegel, K.F.: Foundations of dialectical psychology (Klett, Stuttgart/Academic Press, New York 1979).
Sears, R.: Your ancients revisited: a history of child development; in Hetherington, Review of child development research, vol. 5 (University of Chicago Press, Chicago 1975).
Senn, M.J.E.: Insights on the child development movement in the United States. Monogr. 40, serial No. 161, pp. 3–4 (Society for Research in Child Development, 1975).

Deanna Kuhn
John A. Meacham

Changing Conceptions of the Philosophy of Science and the Foundations of Developmental Psychology

Richard F. Kitchener[1]

Colorado State University, Fort Collins, Colo., USA

Logical positivism, or logical empiricism as it sometimes was called, is perhaps the most well-known philosophy of science in the 20th century. There are signs that *Kuhn's* philosophy of science [*Gutting,* 1980; *Kuhn,* 1962] is replacing logical positivism as the currently most widely read and discussed philosophy of science, but, in psychology at least, logical positivism continues to be the most influential philosophy of science [*Kendler,* 1980; *Turner,* 1967; *Wolman,* 1973]. Sometimes it has this authoritative role explicitly, whereas at other times its presence is felt in an implicit and unconscious way. In either case, however, it continues to provide the philosophical framework underlying much of the current discussion of meta-theoretical issues in psychology and constitutes the justification for the inviolable role given to empirical research in psychology. This influence persists even though psychologists [*Arnold,* 1976; *Gergen,* 1979; *Koch,* 1964; *Weimer,* 1979] continue to criticize this movement and its grip upon psychology. *Koch* [1964, p. 5], for example, has criticized psychologists for failing to keep up with developments in the philosophy of science and instead becoming fixated on a 1930 version of positivism: 'Psychology is thus in the unenviable position of standing on philosophical foundations which began to be vacated by philosophy almost as soon as the former had borrowed them.' The 1950 version of logical positivism, for example, is

---

[1] I wish to thank *Karen Strohm Kitchener* for reading this manuscript and for making many helpful suggestions.

so radically different from the logical positivism of 1930 that one could say, without exaggeration, that it throws into doubt the implicit philosophy of science held by many contemporary psychologists.

Although many developmentalists would insist that developmental psychology has escaped the snare of positivism, I will suggest that it has not – at least not completely – and that there is still something like a positivist legacy among many contemporary developmental psychologists. For example, developmental psychology continues to accept positivistic views concerning inductivism and the scientific method, operationism, and the nature of theory and explanation, even though these views have been severely criticized by recent philosophers of science. Moreover, many of these same critics adopt a developmental philosophy of science, an approach that represents an alternative, more adequate foundation for developmental psychology.

20th Century Philosophy of Science

Logical Positivism

Although 20th century philosophy of science[2] [*Brown*, 1979] has evolved through several stages, it can be divided roughly into two eras: the positivistic era (1930–1960) and the post-positivistic era (1960 to the

---

[2] Among most Anglo-Americans, philosophy of science is taken to be analytic in its approach, stressing the conceptual and logical analysis of theories, assumptions and methods of science, often from a linguistic point of view and employing the methods and techniques of formal logic. Only recently has it become evident that there is more to philosophy of science than what is done by Anglo-Americans, and in addition to analytic philosophy of science (Logical Positivism, Popperianism, etc.) one can also refer to a continental philosophy of science (practiced predominantly in Germany and France). This includes Phenomenology (*Husserl, Heidegger, Merleau-Ponty*), Hermeneutics (*Gadamer, Apel*), Dialectics and Critical Theory (*Habermas, Holzkamp*), Constructivism and the Erlangen-Konstanz schools (*Lorenzen*), Structuralism (*Foucault*), French Historical-Critical philosophy of science (*Brunschvicg, Bachelard*), etc. There are few discussions of these continental schools in English [*Gutting,* 1979; *Heelan,* 1979; *Radnitzky,* 1973], especially in relation to psychology. There are, however, several such discussions in German [*Rombach,* 1974; *Schneewind,* 1977; *Seiffert,* 1978]. There are also good discussions and anthologies in English of several of these individual schools [*Kockelmans and Kisiel,* 1970]. Fortunately there are signs of a new rapprochement between continental and analytic philosophy of science. In the remainder of this paper, however, 'philosophy of science' will refer only to analytic philosophy of science.

present). For the purposes of this paper, the most important differences between these two schools concern a meta-philosophical question: What should the philosophy of science be?

Positivistic philosophy of science can be characterized by several terms: *formalism, Platonism, logicism,* and *prescriptivism.* Using the techniques of mathematical logic, positivism attempted to formalize the underlying logical structure of finished and completed scientific theories (the final products). Being committed to logicism (the view that all philosophical questions are really questions of logic), it maintained that philosophy dealt only with the underlying logical structure or form of a scientific theory or an explanation. The positivists tended to assume there was something called *the* underlying logical form of, for example, a theory, and that all theories shared this same form. As such, this logicism tended to spill over into a Platonism (the assumption that logical structures are real, independent and objective, but also fixed and ideal) and hence that these structures are transcendent of actual examples in the concrete world of flux and change. The task of the philosopher of science, therefore, was to discover this underlying logical form.

As a result of this logicism and Platonism, the positivists had a permanent fear of psychologism (the view that logic was reducible to psychology, and hence that logical questions could be decided by psychological research). They maintained, by contrast, that questions of logical validity could not be decided by factual, psychological investigations [a point that even *Piaget* admits: *Kitchener*, 1980b], and even went so far as to argue that psychology was totally irrelevant to logic and epistemology and hence that all psychological questions were irrelevant to the philosophy of science. This sharp distinction between psychology and logic, in turn, led to the famous distinction between the context of discovery and the context of justification [*Reichenbach*, 1938], i.e. the distinction between the origin, cause or genesis of an idea or hypothesis and the testing of such an idea with respect to its validity and adequacy.

All of this added up to a very 'logical' view of the philosophy of science, but this conception of science was, like all Platonisms, a relatively fixed and static one. There was no consideration, for example, of the growth and development of science (at least as a process), since the valid parts of this process could be captured, it was assumed, in terms of the logical differences between two frozen time-slices of science.

One of the most important consequences of this positivistic conception of the philosophy of science immediately emerges when one considers the obvious question of how these ideal logical models are supposed to apply to real science and scientific practice. Since concrete science often fails to match these formal models, such models appear to be ideals of what a good (or valid) theory, explanation, etc. ought to be. Hence logical positivism tended to become largely prescriptive with respect to scientific concepts and practice.

Post-Positivistic Philosophy of Science
By contrast, contemporary post-positivistic philosophy of science is essentially developmental in its approach. Although there is considerable disagreement among members of this school (*Popper, Lakatos, Kuhn, Feyerabend, Toulmin, Shapere, McMullin*, etc.) there is also substantial agreement. They agree, for example, that an adequate philosophy of science must be evaluated against real (actual) science, both as practiced today and as it has historically evolved. Philosophy of science should not be prescriptive, therefore, but rather must be assessed against real science. Post-positivistic philosophy of science, therefore, tends to be much more descriptive of and empirical about science.

A central problem for the new philosophy of science is the growth and development of science. Fundamental questions concern, for example, the dynamics of theory development, the progress of science, and a new conception of scientific rationality. This, in turn, marks a departure from Platonism, logicism and formalism, towards *historicism* (the view that the nature of, e.g. a theory can only be fully understood by tracing its historical development), *contextualism* (the view that an issue or question must always be raised and answered with respect to its particular and detailed contextual setting) and a stress on *praxis* (goal-directed and theory-guided practice).

As a result, serious doubts are raised about the time-honored distinction between the context of discovery and the context of justification and the positivists' dismissal of psychology (and sociology) as irrelevant to the philosophy of science. The possibility is thus opened up that psychology (especially developmental psychology) may have an important contribution to make to the philosophy of science. For example, there may be important similarities, as *Piaget* points out, between the development of science and individual development [*Kitchener*, 1981, 1982d].

Inductivism

What is the philosophy of science underlying contemporary developmental psychology and what should it be? Four views, typical of positivism, can be found in contemporary developmental psychology: inductivism, operationism, a formalistic model of scientific theories, and the deductive-nomological account of explanation.

Inductivism is a view concerning scientific method characteristically found among 19th century positivists, but it was a tempting view even for 20th century positivists to take and one easily justified by their empiricist epistemology.

Observation

An essential feature of positivist epistemology relates to the foundation of knowledge. According to this view, all scientific knowledge is based upon objective scientific evidence (facts), and scientific facts consist of empirical observations of public spatio-temporal objects. Such observations were said to be the certain (indubitable) basis for everything else and thus represented the foundations of knowledge.

The positivists held a very distinctive view about the nature of (scientific) observation, a view absolutely essential to methodological behaviorism [*Kendler*, 1980; *Kendler and Spence*, 1971; *Kimble*, 1967]: *observations are free of theory*. According to this view, observations are logically prior to and superior to theory, because observations involve no interpretation, inference, conjecture or theoretical bias.

Scientists, according to this view, simply open their eyes and directly (non-inferentially) observe what is directly and immediately present to their senses. No interpretations of inferences 'beyond what is immediately given' (the data) are involved in observing something, and to allow such theoretical interpretations into one's observation (or data language) would be to contaminate a neutral observation (or observation report). All scientists, even of very different theoretical persuasions, see the same things in the same neutral way, namely as their senses directly record input from the environmental objects.

A scientist's particular theory or theoretical interpretation is logically secondary, since observations are supposed to be free of theory. Therefore, when theorists disagree about things, they are disagreeing about the correct interpretation of these antecedent neutral observations. Since these theoretical interpretations constitute a step subsequent to observation, one could either refrain from theorizing because theories are, à la *Skinner* [1950], in principle avoidable or because theories are no more than convenient (conventional) abbreviations of observable functional relations (operational definitions, intervening variables) and hence ultimately reducible to observations. Theoretical disputes are thus merely a question of preference for labels; the 'real' disputes are always about the data.

Inductive Scientific Method

The above view, quickly abandoned by the logical positivists, provides the basis for what can be called *the inductive scientific method*. According to this view, scientific method consists of three steps: first, the collection of observable data; second, the formation of scientific regularities, generalizations and laws, which are inductive generalizations and abstractions from this data; and, finally, the formation of theories, which consist merely of collections of these earlier laws and perhaps include terms which are convenient abbreviations for the lower-level data.

I think a model of science very similar to this lies at the heart of much of contemporary developmental psychology. This seems obviously true in the case of the operant approach [*Bijou and Baer*, 1978], since it is modelled on *Skinner's* operant paradigm, which is explicitly committed to this inductive model [*Kitchener*, 1982b; *Skinner*, 1938, 1947]. But such an approach is also implicitly present in and underlies much of the empirical research done in developmental psychology, research the function of which seems to be largely collection of facts about various aspects of development. Data collection seems widely assumed to be the first and essential step in producing scientific knowledge. Such 'neutral' data are based upon theory-free scientific observation and constitute the secure basis for the much later generation of laws and regularities concerning development. Someday these laws may even provide the basis for a theory of development, which (of course) is in the far-off future. Such a conception, admittedly tacit, seems to characterize the general outlook of many of the research journals in developmental psychology, which stress data collection. Such a view can also be found explicitly in the writings of developmentalists. The following comment, for example, is rather typical:

'It can be seen in this volume that progress has been made and that the student of aging today is in a better position because he (1) has more facts available, (2) has more reliable and more different ways of securing data, and (3) has the beginnings of theory to help organize his information, and through familiarity and training he attains more precision in his statements about problems. Research on aging is undergoing a metamorphosis into an experimental field and, as the facts about aging increase, more and more attention will be given to method and theory not only to manage and systematize the increasing data but also to save time in devising more experiments' [*Birren*, 1959, p. 4].

Likewise, *Baltes* et al. [1977, p. 28] say 'Thus, the scientific method includes obtaining observations in a particular way, generalizing from these observations to the general case, and integrating these generalizations.' Other developmentalists [*Gewirtz*, 1969, pp. 9, 15; *Lerner*, 1976, pp. 4–6; *McCandless and Spiker*, 1956; *Thomas*, 1979, pp. 2, 3, 11] seem to agree with such a model, although several developmentalists are also critical of it [*Baltes* et al., 1977; *Overton*, 1976].

In reply to the claim that these and similiar remarks about 'data collection' are inductivist, it might be said that they are not meant to be taken in an inductivist sense; in fact the standard experimental research paradigm in developmental psychology is incompatible with this inductivist conception. An essential component of this paradigm is first the formulation of experimental hypotheses, which are then tested in the experiment (or quasi-experiment). Thus, so this line of reasoning goes, experimentation really follows something like the hypothetico-deductive model, rather than the inductivist model.

It is certainly true that developmentalists [*Achenbach*, 1978; *Baldwin*, 1960, 1967; *Baltes* et al., 1977] speak of 'testing a hypothesis', and this may lead one to think that data are collected subsequent to this initial hypothesis formation. There is something of merit and importance in this reply. But I think it is still unclear whether it convincingly shows that inductivism is not prevalent in developmental psychology.

First of all, it is not clear what is meant by the hypothetico-deductive method. For example, some psychologists [*Cattell*, 1966; *Marx*, 1963] claim that in the 'hypothetico-deductive method', the hypothesis is really 'induced' from the data, so that the initial step of the hypothetico-deductive method is clearly an inductive one. This interpretation of the hypothetico-deductive method, therefore, is really an inductive-deductive two-step process and can be contrasted with the view [*Popper*, 1965] that where the hypothesis comes from is not important, since the initial starting point is the hypothesis itself and not data. Discussions of the hypothetico-deductive model typically do not make clear which of these two views is meant, even though it is of major importance.

Secondly, it is unclear whether hypotheses are really necessary in scientific research, or whether this is merely a matter of convention. Is there, for example, some epistemological reason that hypotheses are necessary, or do researchers use them merely because they must do so if they are to use the standard statistical models? Standard experimental hypothesis testing via statistical models requires an experimental hypothesis because the statistical model in question typically requires a null hypothesis that (hopefully) will be rejected. But if researchers had a choice between testing a hypothesis and not doing so (as in the operant paradigm), would they continue to do so, and if so why? Suppose, for example, one takes the following position:

> 'Theoretical concepts and assumptions guide the goals, choice of variables, procedures, methods of analysis, and conclusions of all research. Whether a researcher divides the subject matter of development into stimuli and response, instinctual drives and defenses, cognitive structures, or fixed action patterns, he is imposing categories that will dictate his choice of data, the questions he asks of his data, and the types of answers he can obtain. In short any study of development begins with a set of assumptions on the part of the researcher' [*Achenbach*, 1978, p. 19].

Suppose these assumptions have what I will call a strong epistemological function. We would be claiming something more than just that hypotheses have a *directive* function (of telling one where to look among the data and what to focus one's attention on), and more than a *selective* function (of picking out certain kinds of data from a larger array of already existing data). According to this view, our data are not already there in reality waiting for us to collect them, analyze them, and later interpret them. (This is what might be called the archaeological model of data collection.) On the contrary, if our hypotheses play a strong epistemological role, then the very *existence, description* and *meaning* of the data are partly dependent upon our hypotheses. If so, then the assumption that data are permanent and theories transitory must be given up. Why this is so is revealed more clearly by considering a different epistemological view of the nature of scientific observation.

Observations Are 'Theory-Laden'

According to this view, made popular by *Hanson* [1958], *Kuhn* [1962], *Popper* [1965] and others, observations are never totally free of theory and 'pure'. One cannot observe anything unless one first has something like a theory. A theory makes sense out of one's observations, it determines the meaning and significance of what is observed and it literally structures one's observation. Thus, the very existence and meaning of an observable fact logically depends upon a prior theory. According to this view, therefore, two scientists can look at the 'same' thing but see very different things and, in fact, what one literally sees is partly a function of one's cognitive-linguistic-scientific theory. Hence, observation is never neutral and atheoretical, nor is it direct, immediate and non-inferential. On the contrary, observation is always laden with theory.

If we accept this interpretation of observation, it follows that even the best datum is fallible. Based as it is upon a particular theory (e.g. Galileo's telescopic observation of the moon was based upon theories concerning his instrument, optics, physiology [*Feyerabend*, 1975]), this datum or fact may be overturned by another (later) competing theory and this 'fact' declared spurious. A later theory, with hindsight, may claim that earlier 'facts' were impossible, that the observer did not (and could not) observe what he or she claims to have observed, since, for example, there are no such things to be observed (e.g. witches, homunculi in zygotes). Likewise, earlier observers may have been in error in what they observed (or in their data collection) because of some unknown confounding variable, methodological flaw in their design, etc. Facts are not, therefore, infallible building blocks for future laws and theories, since no observational data are infallible and certain. Some developmentalists [*Lerner*, 1976, pp. 3, 4] do admit that earlier 'facts' may be overturned, but (according to them) overturned by new facts, which disprove or correct the earlier 'facts'. But then, of course, these new facts, in turn, may be overruled and corrected by still newer facts, etc. All facts continue to be fallible.

This theory-laden view of observation (unlike its opponent) has the good fortune of being well-supported by psychological knowledge concerning perception and cognition. One of the ironies of methodological behaviorism [*Kendler and Spence*, 1971] and its assumption that scientific observation is neutral and free of all interpretation was that it had to fly in the face of psychological knowledge (e.g. Gestalt psychology) concerning the very psychological nature of observation. It gave the scientist the humanly impossible task of observing something without any prior cognitive structuring or interpretation. But then, of course, methodological behaviorism never took the psychology of perception seriously!

If we were to take this new view of scientific observation seriously, we would view our experimental data in a quite different (fallible) way: we would not consider theory as an end result that some day will emerge from our currently theory-free data and organize them in a coherent, meaningful way. Rather theory would be regarded as being involved from the very start and as permitting us to observe what we do observe. If this view were accepted, therefore, theory would be accorded much more attention and importance than at present.

The claim that developmentalists are primarily concerned with data collection has been disputed by *Bronfenbrenner* [1963], *Looft* [1972], and *Mussen* [1970]. According to them, data collection was characteristic of an earlier period (1930–1960) of developmental psychology but today (i.e. 1960–1970) there is more of a concern with abstract psychological processes, inferred processes, behavioral constructs and, in general, with an explanation of developmental changes, i.e. 'the mechanisms and processes accounting for growth and development' [*Mussen*, 1970, p. vii]. *Mussen* [1970, p. viii] even concludes that theory is more prominent today (i.e. 1970) than it was in 1950.

Although these statements seem correct as far as they go, the question is one of relative degree: There is (perhaps) more theorizing today than before, but data collection is still the dominant theme among many developmentalists, as other developmentalists concede [*Birren*, 1959, 1960]. What these remarks highlight, however, is the need for a more detailed discussion of the nature of theory and explanation in developmental psychology, and especially the conceptual status of these inferred entities and constructs. These are matters that many developmentalists continue to view in a positivistic way.

Operationism

Operational Definitions
A crucial issue in the philosophy of science is the nature of concept formation in the sciences [*Hempel*, 1952]. How should scientific concepts (theoretical constructs, hypothetical terms, etc.) be introduced into science? What criteria must they satisfy? Must they, for example, be given definitions or only partial meanings? Must their definitions be empirical?

After an initial suggestion that *all* theoretical constructs should be explicitly defined in terms of observable properties, the early positivists suggested that *all scientific concepts must be operationally defined.* As originally understood [*Hempel*, 1954; *Stevens*, 1939], this thesis of operationism claimed that the complete and total meaning of a concept was to be given by the operations performed by the experimenter and the results observed. This (it was claimed) is what the concept of 'length' means, namely the result of measuring an object by some yardstick.

This doctrine has had a very checkered and controversial history, especially in psychology [*Bergmann and Spence*, 1941; *Feigl*, 1945; *Hempel*, 1954; *Stevens*, 1939]. As a thesis concerning scientific concept formation, it was subjected to a series of radical criticisms beginning with *Carnap's* [1936–37] early and most famous criticism [see *Hempel* 1952, 1965a, and *Koch*, 1964, for a history of these criticisms]. By 1950, such a view had been abandoned by the logical positivists (the one exception is *Bergman* [1957], who has continued undauntedly to espouse operationism; his devoted students at Iowa, especially in psychology, have continued to follow his lead) in favor of much more liberal criteria involving 'open' hypothetical constructs anchored much less securely to empirical data. These ties were progressively weakened so that, by 1970, even these more liberal interpretations of how constructs are related to data were abandoned [*Hempel*, 1970].

The evolution and eventual abandonment of operationism has not been reflected in contemporary developmental psychology (or psychology at large). Numerous developmentalists from strikingly different theoretical camps insist that theoretical constructs should be 'operationally defined' and 'operationalized' [*Achenbach*, 1978, pp. 75, 76; *Baltes* et al., 1977, pp. 28, 66, 80; *Birren*, 1959, p. 11; *Birren and Renner*, 1977, pp. 13, 24; *Bromley*, 1970, pp. 86, 95; *Gewirtz*, 1969; *Lerner*, 1976, p. 293; *McCandless and Spiker*, 1956; *Reese and Overton*, 1970, p. 116].

Of course, many developmentalists might respond that they do not mean by 'operational definition' what positivist philosophers meant. They do not mean, that is, that every theoretical construct should be operationally defined in the strict sense, only that experimental (empirical) variables that are being used as a test of a theory, as a measurement, or as an empirical indicator of a theory must be 'operationalized'. One must specify how to translate such a variable into experimental or quasi-experimental terms, i.e. one must specify the operations to be performed. On this account, therefore, operationism is a thesis valid in the context of research designed to test some theory [*Achenbach*, 1978; *Lerner*, 1976], but it is not meant to apply to the context of theory construction and elaboration [*Baldwin*, 1960, 1967].

Whether 'operationism' is meant in the strict or loose sense (and it is typically unclear which interpretation an author is employing), the term tends to be seriously misleading. Historically, operationism has been a distinctive and controversial thesis (at least in its strong form) that arose in a particular context and had a precise meaning. When it is used in a different (weaker) sense, the shift in meaning is not always noted, nor consistently followed. The result, therefore, is often conceptual confusion, in which 'operationism' is used as a weapon against a theoretical opponent.

This point can perhaps be most clearly seen in the now classic criticism of *Piaget's* stage theory by *Brainerd* [1978]. His criticisms of *Piaget's* stage theory clearly presuppose positivism, behaviorism and operationism. According to *Brainerd* [1978, pp. 174, 209] in order for something to be a legitimate explanatory construct, it must fulfill three conditions; (1) it 'must specify some target behaviors that undergo change', (2) it must posit or specify antecedent variables believed to be causally responsible for such changes in behavior (these variables presumably being 'maturational and experiential'), and (3) 'procedures whereby the antecedent variables can be measured *independently* of behavioral changes must also be specified'.

These three conditions clearly show two things. First, *Brainerd* [1978] is insisting that a legitimate explanatory construct must be operationally defined. Hence it must become an intervening variable: Once one specifies the consequent behavior and the antecedent variable responsible for it, one has specified what the entire construct is. What else is the construct, over and above these antecedent-consequent relations? Clearly, his conditions are tantamount to insisting that a cognitive (stage) structure (the particular explanatory construct of concern to *Brainerd*) be merely an intervening variable, one to be operationally defined. But such a request is based upon an archaic and untenable conception of the philosophy of science.

Secondly, his requirements clearly show what he takes an explanation to be, for it is the antecedent variable(s) that are causally responsible for the consequent behavior and hence do the explaining. If these antecedent conditions do the explaining, however, what explanatory role is left for a stage structure? Clearly none. This comes out clearly in *Kurtines'* [1978] comments on *Brainerd's* position:

> '*Brainerd's* second criterion (i.e. that a theory posit antecedent variables, which I take to mean some sort of plausible explanatory variables or causal mechanism that are at least in principle capable of operational definition) seems to be a reasonable enough theoretical requirement, and in itself provides the basis for a potentially powerful critique of most current stage theories...'
>
> 'A more powerful criticism of the current proliferation of stage models, I would like to suggest, is that *they lack explanatory power because they fail to specify any plausible explanatory variables at all*' [p. 193, my italics].

There is thus a subtle temptation to move from insisting that one give an operational definition of one's research variables or those empirical conditions that might constitute a test of one's theoretical construct to the conclusion that such independent-dependent variables *are* (or should be) the theoretical construct, and hence that the real explanation consists of these antecedent (typically environmental) variables that cause the consequent behavior. Hence, on this account, there could be no explanatory causal mechanism at all that was not itself operationally definable. If an explanatory construct were not operationally definable, it would lack any explanatory power.

Hypothetical Constructs and Beyond

These positivistic structures of *Brainerd* (and others) are thus tantamount to the claim that *all theoretical constructs must be no more than intervening variables* [*Tolman*, 1936] and hence that no hypothetical constructs [*MacCorquodale and Meehl*, 1948] should be allowed. But, once again, to countenance only intervening variables is to adopt a philosophy of science that was outmoded already at the time of the classic *MacCorquodale and Meehl* [1948] distinction. As the subsequent history of positivism clearly shows, philosophers of science became convinced that intervening variables, because theoretically expendable, have no theoretical, explanatory power [*Braithwaite*, 1953] and that, consequently, hypothetical constructs are a more powerful theoretical device.

The logic of hypothetical constructs (as opposed to intervening variables) constitutes a distinctive brand of theory construction, involving nomological networks, open concepts, multiple (probabilistic) indicators, and 'converging operations' [*Campbell and Fiske*, 1959;

Cronbach and Meehl, 1955; *Garner* et al., 1956; *Hempel*, 1952; *Kaplan*, 1946; *Pap*, 1953]. But one of the essential features of such hypothetical constructs is their 'surplus meaning', their 'openness' and their less secure empirical ties. However, the most powerful explanatory constructs in science (e.g. atom, electron, field, gene, germ) seem to have precisely these same properties. The scientific payoff is thus explanatory power over empirical certainty.

The logic of hypothetical constructs, however, proved to be too restrictive and soon gave way to a new interest in the role and power of theoretical models in science, leading to a thoroughly non-positivistic conception of models [*Achinstein*, 1958; *Harre*, 1972; *Hesse*, 1966]. According to this view, models no longer have, as in positivism, merely a heuristic role [*Baltes and Willis*, 1977; *Baltes* et al., 1977], but rather play a key explanatory role. Models are postulated, unobservable hidden structures or 'generative mechanisms' that explain observable phenomena [*Harre*, 1972; *McMullin*, 1978]. As such, models play an essential theoretical role in science and function in ways very similar to those proposed by *Piaget* [1968, 1973] with respect to the nature of scientific explanation. If this approach to models is taken seriously, it would, contra many developmentalists such as *Brainerd* [1978], involve the notion of 'hidden structures' that play the fundamental theoretical role in scientific explanation.

For our purposes what is important is not a detailed recounting of all the developments that have occurred in 20th century philosophy of science concerning the nature of concept formation. More important to note are some of the reasons underlying these developments, especially in the case of operationism.

If a scientist were to operationally define every theoretical concept in such a way that the meaning of this concept were fixed by observations, it would be stultifying to scientific progress (especially scientific explanation). If we look to scientific practice, we find that the meaning of a concept is not exhaustively given at any one point in time, but rather changes as a function of new empirical knowledge [*Baltes* et al., 1977, p. 4]. The best scientific theorizing (e.g. in physics) is thus dynamic and continually developing. A concept often is introduced initially with a very unclear meaning and, as research progresses, its meaning is progressively tied down to the empirical domain. Hence, a construct is progressively modified and takes on new meaning as a function of empirical research. The rationale underlying this process is the explanatory role such constructs are supposed to perform, a role that necessitates their hypothetical character. As *Hempel* [1965a, pp. 205, 206] puts it:

'... when a scientist introduces theoretical entities such as electric currents, magnetic fields, chemical valencies, or subconscious mechanisms, he intends them to serve as explanatory factors which have an existence independent of the observable symptoms by which they manifest themselves; or, to put it in more sober terms: whatever observational criteria of application the scientist may provide are intended by him to describe just symptoms or indications of the presence of the entity in question, but not to give an exhaustive characterization of it. The scientist does indeed wish to leave open the possibility of adding to this theory further statements involving his theoretical terms – statements which may yield new interpretative connections between theoretical and observational terms; and yet he will regard these as additional assumptions about the same hypothetical entities to which the theoretical terms referred before the expansion. This way of looking at theoretical terms appears to have definite heuristic value. It stimulates the invention and use of powerfully explanatory concepts for which only some links with experience can be indicated at the time, but which are fruitful in suggesting further lines of research that may lead to additional connections with the data of direct observation.'

A construct is thus 'open' in terms of its meaning and explanatory power and has a kind of historical life of its own, proceeding according to what can be called a developmental (even dialectical) logic. This conception suggests obvious parallels with cognitive developmental psychology and with good reason, for the formation and development of concepts in science is (partly at least) a human cognitive activity. It is only to be expected, therefore, that a theory about the development of concepts in the individual will have something to contribute toward clarifying the development of concepts in the scientist.

Theory

Theories as Formal Systems Partially Interpreted
As the preceding discussion has revealed, the nature of scientific concepts is a topic that has had a rich and diverse history. The logical positivists' conception of a theory, by contrast, changed very little from 1930 to 1960. Committed as they were to a formalistic ideal, the positivists believed the best way to understand the nature of scientific theories was to conceptualize them from a logical, formal point of view, i.e. to imagine that a scientific theory had an underlying implicit

formal-logical structure and that the most adequate and precise scientific theories (e.g. *Newton's*) could be axiomatized into a formal geometrical system. This at least was the ideal toward which all theories eventually should aspire and the one that some psychologists (such as *Hull*) explicitly adapted.

According to this view, scientific theories consisted of a set of uninterpreted axioms, definitions and rules of inference. Theoretical terms were said to be 'implicitly defined' by this set of axioms. In addition, a set of principles (variously called coordinating definitions, operational definitions, correspondence principles, epistemic correlations, bridge principles, etc.) was required that related these formal, theoretical components to the empirical world and gave them their semantic meaning and empirical reference. Such coordinating definitions provided for the 'partial interpretation' of one's theoretical terms [*Hempel*, 1952, 1965a; *Suppe*, 1974].

For our purposes, two aspects of this 'received view' are especially important: (1) According to this view, a correspondence rule 'specifies the meaning of the terms only *partially* and thus does not provide a way of eliminating the term from all contexts in which it may occur' [*Hempel*, 1965a, p. 296]. Hence, it 'treats theoretical concepts as "open"' [p. 189]. (2) Such correspondence rules or coordinating 'definitions' give only a *partial* interpretation of *some* of the theoretical terms in a theory: '... it does not lay down for every term in [one's theory], a necessary and sufficient condition of application' [*Hempel*, 1965a, p. 209]. In fact, 'it is quite possible that an interpretative system provides, for some or even *all* of the terms in (our theoretical system), no necessary or no sufficient condition in terms of (our basic observational language), or indeed neither of the two' [*Hempel*, 1965a, p. 210, my italics]. Raising these technical points is important in order to see what was really meant by 'coordinating definitions', a point that will emerge again when we discuss how developmentalists use the terms 'theory' and 'coordinating definition'.

In a less formalistic way, one could also say that a theory consisted of a set of laws (e.g. *Newton's* laws of mechanics and gravitation), but this expression was understood to be merely a more convenient way of referring to the structure of a theory, which was to be more fully explicated as an axiomatic system. Such a view of theory (as a collection of empirical laws) fit in quite nicely with the early positivists' inductivist epistemology in which one first collected facts, then induced more general laws, and finally added several of these laws together to form a theory.

Theory in Developmental Psychology

When the nature of theory is discussed in developmental psychology, the preceding interpretation is often to be found. *Baltes and Willis* [1977, pp. 129, 130], for example, say: 'Scientific theories form a deductive system. A theory is a set of statements including (a) general laws and principles that serve as axioms or assumptions, (b) other laws which are deductible from the general axioms, and (c) coordinating definitions relating theoretical terms to observational sentences.' Such a view is not uncommon [*Baltes* et al., 1977; *Baltes and Cornelius*, 1977; *Baldwin*, 1960, 1967; *Bromley*, 1970; *Gewirtz*, 1969; *McCandless and Spiker*, 1956; *Reese and Overton*, 1970]. Likewise, the basic axioms of a scientific theory are typically thought to consist of empirical laws describing observable phenomena. For example, *Baltes* et al. [1977, pp. 16, 17] say: 'In science, a theory is a set of statements including (1) laws and (2) definitions of terms. The laws of science, or principles of science, are statements about relationships between variables' such as Boyle's law and the law of least effort. Such a view becomes unavoidable if one assumes that all theoretical terms must be given operational definitions (coordinating definitions), as most of these authors do.

But, as we have just seen, to claim that a theoretical system must be given a partial interpretation in terms of correspondence rules did not mean that such correspondence rules were operational definitions (or that they were really definitions at all), nor did it mean that *each* theoretical term must be given a 'coordinating definition', as *Baltes* et al. [1977] apparently think. For example, *Gewirtz* [1969, p. 10] criticizes theories of socialization for not emphasizing 'operational definitions underlying their empirical terms, explicit definitions of their theoretical terms, nor coordinating definitions between theoretical and empirical terms that specify unambiguously the circumstances under which theoretical terms are to be used (i.e. their referents).' But, as we have seen, none of these three conditions is necessary *even according to the positivists*.

This point is especially crucial when we consider the claim [*Baltes and Cornelius*, 1977; *Baltes* et al., 1980; *Lerner* et al., 1980] that all theories and paradigms must abide by 'the scientific method', which allegedly is neutral with respect to different theoretical frameworks (e.g. behaviorism versus dialectics). Although it is not clear what the scientific method is, nor whether there is only one, *Baltes* et al. [1977] seem to equate the scientific method with the experimental (and quasi-experimental) research paradigms current in experimental psychology, or sometimes [*Baltes and Cornelius*, 1977, p. 127] even more explicitly with logical positivism, since 'the *scientific method*... involves primarily... the formulation of coordinating definitions relating theoretical terms to observational sentences.' As we have just seen, this view of the nature of a theory was explicitly a positivistic one and is no longer considered valid, much less sacrosanct. Likewise, in light of the current disputes over the scientific method itself, it is surprising to read: '...Well-established procedures for verification or falsification and proof are generalizable across all such world views' [*Lerner* et al., 1980, p. 227]. This is especially questionable since, as *Rappoport* [1980] correctly points out, 'established positivistic research methods are dialectically embedded in the deep structure of contemporary psychology'. The requirement that all paradigms abide by 'the scientific method', therefore, is really the requirement that dialectics, for example, must abide by a positivistic epistemology with respect to theory construction.

Non-Positivistic Views of Theory

There is little doubt that some scientific theories can be interpreted as formal theories and can be axiomatized. The real question, however, is whether this is the fundamental sense of 'theory' or whether there are other notions of theory that are equally plausible and more enlightening for developmental psychology.

Several philosophers of science have challenged the positivistic notion of a formalized theory [*Achinstein*, 1968; *Hanson*, 1958; *Kaplan*, 1964; *Lakatos*, 1970; *Suppe*, 1974; *Toulmin*, 1953, 1961], including *Hempel* [1970] himself. The most decisive objection to this formal model of scientific theories is one that we have already touched upon, one that should be especially compelling to developmentalists. The formal model of a scientific theory takes the end products of scientific research, the static and finished products present in a momentary, frozen time-slice, as definitive and essential for what a scientific theory is (and should be). It takes a 'snapshot' of a theory and maintains that this is the entire theory. But what this synchronic approach ignores is the obvious fact that a theory is not a static and fixed, momentary entity, but rather a dynamic and evolving entity. It is an entity that has a history of changes such that to understand it, one must understand this dynamic development, i.e. the changes that occurred in the theory and why they occurred.

As *McMullin* [1970, p. 14] put it:

> 'It is not enough for the philosopher to consider a 'slice' of scientific work at a moment in time. Rather, he has to trace the sequences by which concepts are gradually modified in the course of time, the way in which the fertility of a hypothesis over the course of time serves to confirm its validity, and the manner in which a model can continue to guide research over a long period of time so that one can legitimately suppose it to provide an approximate insight into the real structure of the object studied.'

Such a view clearly involves taking a diachronic perspective and treating a theory as a developmental entity.

But if a theory is not just a frozen time-slice of logical relations, but rather a dynamic developmental entity composed of stages, it is also a *whole*, with an underlying *structure* to it. A theory is not a simple, atomistic conjunction of empirical laws; it is a structured whole in which the relations between the parts are not simple conjunctions [*Kitchener*, 1982a].

This holistic view of theories has been expressed by several philosophers of science, but by none perhaps so clearly as *Kuhn* [1977, pp. 19, 20]:

> 'Theories, as the historian knows them, cannot be decomposed into constituent elements for purposes of direct comparison either with nature or with each other. That is not to say that they cannot be analytically decomposed at all, but rather that the lawlike parts produced by analysis cannot, unlike empirical laws, function individually in such comparisons.'

Hence, theories 'are clearly unlike laws' in the way they function and in the way they are tested and evaluated [*Kuhn*, 1977, p. 20].

According to at least some post-positivistic philosophers of science, therefore, theories are seen both as structured wholes and as possessing a developmental history. Once more, some convergence appears between contemporary philosophy of science and cognitive developmental psychology.

Explanation

The Deductive-Nomological Model

One of the most characteristic theses of logical empiricism concerned the nature of scientific explanation. According to the classic account of *Hempel* [1965b], an explanation of a fact consists of a set of laws and antecedent conditions from which the fact in question can be deduced. Likewise, the explanation of a law consists of a set of laws from which the particular law in question can be deduced. Hence, 'all explanation is deduction', and thus this model was called the *deductive-nomological* model.

A famous corollary of this view of explanation was the *symmetry thesis*: explanation and prediction are symmetrical concepts. The only difference between them is one of temporal order. In an explanation, we have a fact to be explained first and the explanation is provided afterwards, whereas in a prediction, we have a set of laws and antecedent conditions first and the derived prediction second. To explain something is thus equivalent to predicting it and to predict something is equivalent to explaining it.

This model applies most clearly to the case of a causal explanation. The antecedent conditions, for example, can typically be construed as the cause of the fact to be explained. The laws themselves (according to early versions of this model) would most likely be cause-effect relationships involving observable, antecedent-consequent variables (or perhaps more complex laws involving the micro-structure of an object). These antecedent conditions (together with the laws) would thus causally explain the effect and, as a sufficient condition for the effect, they would allow one to predict and control the effect at will.

This model of explanation seems closely tied to the experimental paradigm in psychology, in which the dependent variable (behavior) is a function of independent variables (manipulable, environmental variables). It is tempting to conclude that since the dependent variable is a function of the independent variable (the independent variable influences [affects] the dependent variable, the independent variable 'accounts for' so much variance in the dependent variable, etc.), then the independent variable is the variable causing the corresponding changes in the dependent variable. This is especially true if you believe, as the early positivists and *Skinner* [1938] do, that causality is merely a functional relation. Thus, if the independent variable is the cause of the behavior, it must be the explanation of that behavior. But if we have a (causal) explanation of the behavior via its environmental antecedents and functional relations (between independent and dependent variables), we obviously have an explanation; nothing else theoretical, hypothetical or observable seems to be needed. Thus, not only is such an experimental model in keeping with the positivistic model of explanation, it seems to be committed to a *methodological behaviorism* [*Achenbach*, 1978; *Ausubel* et al., 1980; *Baltes and Willis*, 1977; *Baltes* et al., 1977, 1980; *Brainerd*, 1978; *Gewirtz*, 1969].

Methodological behaviorism had its home in classical learning theory, especially in the theories of *Hull, Spence* and *Tolman* [*Kitchener*, 1977], and was explicitly based upon the philosophy of logical positivism [*Koch*, 1964]. Given our preceding points, it thus appears odd that developmental psychologists continue to endorse methodological behaviorism as the experimental research paradigm for developmental psychology and even apparently to identify it, as we have seen, with the scientific method.

This endorsement may be due partly to the widespread assumption that developmental psychology is the study of changes in behavior as a function of age or age-correlated causes (e.g. maturation and learning) [*Baltes* et al., 1977]. Thus, an explanation of development will consist of a set of antecedent, independent, experimental variables of which behavior will be a function. As *Baltes* et al. [1977, p. 177] put it: 'In explanatory research, age-change functions or alternative developmental phenomena typically are seen as part of the dependent variable ... and researchers' efforts are aimed at finding the controlling variables and processes.' This naturally leads to thinking about these antecedent-consequent relationships between experimental variables as scientific laws and viewing these antecedent variables as the causes (and hence the explanations) of behavior. Since causes are typically construed as sufficient conditions for a phenomenon, such conditions permit both prediction (knowing the antecedent condition, one can predict the consequent condition) and control (e.g. by producing the sufficient condition one can produce the consequent). In the latter sense, causes are often said to be *handles* or *recipes* for producing effects [*Kitchener*, 1982c].

New Models of Explanation

It is clear, therefore, that many developmentalists subscribe to a model of explanation very similar to the positivist's general deductive-nomological model as well as to the more particular causal form of this model [*Baltes* et al., 1977, p. 28; *Brainerd*, 1978; *Bromley*, 1970, p. 85; *Birren*, 1959, p. 9; *Lerner*, 1976, p. 12; *McCandless and Spiker*, 1956; *Reese and Overton*, 1970]. Again, there is no doubt that some scientific explanations are deductive-nomological in nature and that many explanations involve sufficient conditions. But the real question is whether this is the only kind of legitimate scientific explanation or whether there are alternative (equally legitimate) types of explanations that are perhaps more suitable for the developmental sciences in general and for developmental psychology in particular. As *Baltes* et al. [1977] point out, the developmental sciences (astronomy, archeology, history, biology, geology) share a basic outlook. This similarity in outlook may extend to the kinds of explanations offered. These sciences provide developmental explanations, in contrast to the physical sciences, which are typically non-historical and employ 'process' or causal explanations [*Bergmann*, 1957; *Hempel*, 1965b; *Kitchener*, 1982c; *Mandelbaum*, 1971; *Woodward*, 1980]. Although such developmental explanations may employ *developmental laws*, thus leading some philosophers [*Hempel*, 1965b] to suggest that developmental explanations do conform to the deductive-nomological model, most philosophers seem to believe that even with the inclusion of developmental laws, developmental explanations are not examples of causal deductive nomological explanations. For this reason, many philosophers [*Mandelbaum*, 1961; *Woodward*, 1980] claim that this makes them inadequate as explanations and that someday they will be replaced by (adequate causal) explanations. Others [*Kitchener*, 1982c] have argued that developmental explanations are perfectly good 'as is' and that only positivistic biases lead us to suppose they are inferior. According to this account, developmental explanations are an example of a *pattern explanation* [*Baltes* et al., 1977; *Kaplan*, 1964] and a *how-possibly* explanation [*Dray*, 1957] in which a stage law explains a particular stage by providing a larger structural-functional explanation involving formal and final causes. Thus, as several developmentalists [*Lerner*, 1976; *Overton and Reese*, 1973; *Reese and Overton*, 1970] have argued, developmental explanations are not like the explanations given in the physical sciences but rather represent a distinctive type of explanation. What kind of explanation they are, how they are supposed to explain developmental phenomena, whether they are autonomous or not, etc., are questions still to be resolved.

Contrary to the opinions of some developmentalists and many philosophers, these explanations seem to be both autonomous (non-reducible) and non-causal. Part of the force behind the boldness of such a claim comes from a general waning of confidence in the deductive-nomological model (due to a series of criticisms) and the construction, in turn, of alternative models of explanation, both for the physical sciences and the developmental sciences. For example several philosophers [*Hanson*, 1958; *Scriven*, 1959a] have argued that explanation and prediction are not symmetrical. In the historical-developmental sciences (e.g. evolutionary theory), one can explain but not predict, and, on the other hand, one can often predict something without explaining it (e.g. a score on one test allows one to predict a score on a closely related type of test without the first score being the explanation of the second). In the face of these criticisms, *Hempel* [1965b] has in part abandoned the symmetry thesis.

Likewise, several philosophers [*Scriven*, 1959b] have questioned the assumption that an explanation must contain *laws* at all. It has also been argued that an explanation need not be deductive, nor involve sufficient conditions. Perfectly good explanations (especially in the historical-genetic sciences) often consist merely, so it is claimed, of citing necessary conditions [*Gallie*, 1959] or of giving narrative-type explanations [*Danto*, 1968].

There are thus several different models of explanation presently available to developmentalists. No longer need it be assumed out of hand that all developmental explanations must adhere to the positivistic model. It is at least an open question as to which model of explanation is the most adequate and appropriate model for a developmental explanation: narrative, necessary condition, how-possibly, teleological, deductive-nomological, causal, etc.

Conclusion

20th century philosophy of science has had a dynamic history of change. Beginning with a positivistic philosophy of science that was non-developmental and prescriptive, it gradually changed and became much more developmental in nature, concerned with characterizing science as it really is. As we have seen, several positivistic views, implicit in developmental psychology, either have been abandoned by the positivists themselves or have been successfully challenged and criticized by non-positivistic philosophers of science. These views are essentially static, logicistic, Platonistic, and non-developmental in nature, and thus unsuited for a developmental psychology. Alternative conceptions of these same issues have been advanced by post-positivistic philosophers. Many of these views are developmental in nature or inspired by developmental sciences (including the history of science) and reflect more accurately how scientists really practice science as a dynamically developing, human enterprise. These alternative models are thus more suited to a developmental psychology.

But if developmental psychologists were to take contemporary philosophy of science more seriously, it would not mean that philosophy of science should prescribe or legislate what the foundations of developmental psychology ought to be. Historically, psychologists have given such a role to the philosophy of science and developmentalists have tended to follow suit. It does mean, however, that there are several different models of science, and developmentalists need not (and I would urge ought not) be committed to a positivistic one, especially in the light of the criticisms it has received. The questions rather should be which philosophy of science is conceptually and logically most adequate, and which one is most relevant for a developmental psychology. From my preceding remarks, it is obvious what my own answers to these questions are. But I am not saying that developmentalists should switch models because another philosophy of science is now fashionable and positivism is out of vogue. What I am saying is rather this: There were good reasons why positivism died, and if positivism is to provide the underlying philosophy of science for developmental psychology then the arguments against positivism must be discussed and answered. That may still be possible, and it might turn out that such a neo-positivism (or neo-neo-positivism) would be plausible and adequate. But such a neo-positivism would be very different (and superior) to that popular in the 1950s.

Finally, it should be pointed out that the influence and interaction between philosophy of science and developmental psychology cannot and should not be unidirectional, with developmentalists being influenced by philosophy of science but not the reverse. On the contrary, what the new developmental philosophy of science makes (or should make) clear is that it has equally as much to learn from psychology (including developmental psychology) as psychology has to learn from it.

One of the keynotes of this new historically oriented philosophy of science is a new sense of the relevance of psychology to philosophy of science. This includes not only psychological knowledge about perception and cognition (which, I have suggested, should cast doubt on inductivism), but also, in particular, the areas of concept formation, problem-solving, decision theory, creativity, etc. These areas will prove to be of considerable value and assistance to philosophers concerned with problems of scientific discovery, creativity and rationality. That this is so is already becoming evident to some philosophers [*Nickles*, 1980a, b] as well as psychologists [*Tweney* et al., 1981].

But if psychology is relevant to philosophy of science, the particular branch of psychology that may prove to be most relevant to a developmental or historically oriented philosophy of science is developmental psychology. There are numerous ways in which developmental psychology could make this kind of contribution, but one of the most obvious ones has to do with cognitive development in general, including the development of concepts and categories, the evolution of reasoning skills and styles, the development of problem-solving strategies and heuristics, etc. If the practice of science consists of and depends upon the evolution of certain kinds of cognitive activity in the scientist, it seems obvious that study of the evolution of this kind of cognitive activity in the individual will help us to understand the correlative activity in the scientist and hence the nature of science itself. Although a few developmentalists such as *Piaget* [*Kitchener*, 1980a] and many philosophers [*Toulmin*, 1972] have seen this point clearly, many others have not yet done so.

Summary

Logical positivism continues to be an influential philosophy of science, even in developmental psychology. Four major tenets of logical positivism were selected as examples: (1) a belief in an inductive scientific method together with a sharp distinction between theory and observation, (2) an insistence that all scientific terms be operationally defined, (3) the assumption that a scientific theory has an underlying formal structure, consisting of axioms, definitions, inference rules together with correspondence rules, and (4) the view that a scientific explanation is deductive-nomological in nature. These views, I argue, are still prevalent in contemporary developmental psychology. Several criticisms of these positivistic theses are cited: (a) scientific method is inadequately characterized as inductive in nature and no sharp theory-observation distinction can be made, (b) scientific terms need not be operationally defined but rather are 'open' hypothetical constructs often weakly anchored to experimental data, (c) scientific theories are inadequately characterized as abstract formal entities and instead can better be viewed as holistic, developmental entities, and (d) there are several models of explanation besides the deductive-nomological one, including teleological explanations, developmental explanations, narrative explanations, etc. These alternative, post-positivistic suggestions constitute a more adequate philosophy of science and one more suitable for developmental psychology.

References

Achenbach, T.M.: Research in developmental psychology: concepts, strategies, methods (Free Press, New York 1978).
Achinstein, P.: Concepts of science (Johns Hopkins Press, Baltimore 1968).
Arnold, W.J.: Nebraska symposium on motivation, 1975: conceptual foundations of psychology (University of Nebraska Press, Lincoln 1976).
Ausubel, D.P.; Sullivan, E.V.; Ives, S.W.: Theory and problems of child development; 3rd ed. (Grune & Stratton, New York 1980).
Baldwin, A.L.: The study of child development; in Mussen, Handbook of research methods in child development (Wiley, New York 1960).
Baldwin, A.L.: General issues of behavior theory; in Baldwin, Theories of child development (Wiley, New York 1967).
Baltes, P.; Cornelius, S.W.: The status of dialectics in developmental psychology: theoretical orientation versus scientific method; in Datan, Reese, Life-span developmental psychology: dialectical perspectives on experimental research (Academic Press, New York 1977).
Baltes, P.B.; Reese, H.W.; Lipsitt, L.P.: Life-span developmental psychology. Ann. Rev. Psych. *31:* 65–110 (1980).
Baltes, P.B.; Reese, H.W.; Nesselroade, J.R.: Life-span developmental psychology: introduction to research methods (Brooks/Cole, Monterey 1977).
Baltes, P.B.; Willis, S.L.: Toward psychological theories of aging and human development; in Birren, Schaie, Handbook of the psychology of aging (Van Nostrand Reinhold, New York 1977).
Bergmann, G.: Philosophy of science (University of Wisconsin Press, Madison 1957).
Bergman, G.; Spence, K.: Operationism and theory in psychology. Psych. Rev. *48:* 1–14 (1941).
Bijou, S.W.; Baer, D.M.: Behavior analysis of child development (Prentice-Hall, Englewood Cliffs 1978).
Birren, J.E.: Principles of research on aging, in Birren, Handbook of aging and the individual (University of Chicago Press, Chicago 1959).
Birren, J.E.: Behavioral theories of aging; in Shock, Aging: some social and biological aspects (Am. Association for the Advancement of Science, Washington, 1960).
Birren, J.E.; Renner, V.J.: Research on the psychology of aging; in Birren, Schaie, Handbook of the psychology of aging (Van Nostrand, New York 1977).
Brainerd, C.J.: The stage question in cognitive developmental theory. Behav. Brain Sci. *2:* 173–182 (1978).

Braithwaite, R.: Scientific explanation (Cambridge University Press, Cambridge 1953).

Bromley, D.B.: An approach to theory construction in the psychology of development and aging; in Goulet, Baltes, Life-span developmental psychology: research and theory (Academic Press, New York 1970).

Bronfenbrenner, U.: Developmental theory in transition; in Stevenson, Child psychology. 62nd Yearbook of the National Society for the Study of Education (University of Chicago Press, Chicago 1963).

Brown, H.: Perception, theory and commitment; the new philosophy of science (University of Chicago Press, Chicago 1979).

Campbell, D.T.; Fiske, D.W.: Convergent and discriminant validation by the multitrait-multimethod matrix. Psych. Bull. *56:* 81–105 (1959).

Carnap, R.: Testability and meaning. Phil. Sci. *3:* 420–478; *4:* 1–40 (1936/37).

Cattell, R.B.: Psychological theory and scientific method; in Cattell, Handbook of multivariate experimental psychology (Rand McNally, Chicago 1966).

Cronbach, L.J.; Meehl, P.E.: Construct validity in psychological tests. Psych. Bull. *52:* 281–302 (1955).

Danto, A.: Analytic philosophy of history (Cambridge University Press, New York 1968).

Dray, W.: Law and explanation in history (Oxford University Press, Oxford 1957).

Feigl, H.: Operationism and scientific method, Psych. Rev. *52:* 250–259 (1945).

Feyerabend, P.K.: Against method (NLB, London 1975).

Gallie, W.B.: Explanations in history and the genetic sciences; in Gardiner, Theories of history (Free Press, Glencoe 1959).

Garner, W.R.; Hake, H.W.; Eriksen, C.W.: Operationism and the concept of perception. Psych. Rev. *63:* 149–159 (1956).

Gergen, K.J.: The positivist image in social psychological theory; in Buss, Psychology in social context (Irvington, New York 1979).

Gewirtz, J.L.: Levels of conceptual analysis in environment-infant interaction research. Merrill-Palmer Q. *15:* 7–47 (1969).

Gutting, G.: Continental philosophy of science; in Asquith, Kyburg, Current research in philosophy of science (Philosophy of Science Association, East Lansing 1979).

Gutting, G.: Paradigm and revolutions: applications and appraisals of Thomas Kuhn's philosophy of science (University of Notre Dame Press, Notre Dame 1980).

Hanson, N.R.: Patterns of discovery (Cambridge University Press, Cambridge 1958).

Harre, R.: Principles of scientific thinking (University of Chicago Press, Chicago 1972).

Heelan, P.A.: Continental philosophy and philosophy of science; in Asquith, Kyburg, Current research in the philosophy of science (Philosophy of Science Association, East Lansing 1979).

Hempel, C.G.: Fundamentals of concept formation in the empirical sciences (University of Chicago Press, Chicago 1952).

Hempel, C.G.: A logical appraisal of operationism. Sci. Mon. *79:* 215–220 (1954).

Hempel, C.G.: The theoretician's dilemma: a study in the logic of theory construction; in Hempel, Aspects of scientific explanation (Free Press, New York 1965a).

Hempel, C.G.: Aspects of scientific explanation; in Hempel, Aspects of scientific explanation (Free Press, New York 1965b).

Hempel, C.G.: On the standard conception of scientific theories; in Radner, Winokur, Minnesota studies in the philosophy of science, Vol. IV (University of Minnesota Press, Minneapolis 1970).

Hesse, M.: Models and analogies in science (University of Notre Dame Press, Notre Dame 1966).
Kaplan, A.: Definition and specification of meaning. J. Phil. *43:* 281–288 (1946).
Kaplan, A.: The conduct of inquiry (Chandler, San Francisco 1964).
Kendler, H.H.: Psychology; a science in conflict (Oxford University Press, New York 1980).
Kendler, H.H.; Spence, J.T.: Tenets of neobehaviorism; in Kendler, Spence, Essays in neobehaviorism (Appleton Century Crofts, New York 1971).
Kimble, G.: The basic tenet of behaviorism; in Kimble, Foundations of conditioning and learning (Appleton Century Crofts, New York 1967).
Kitchener, R.F.: B.F. Skinner: the butcher, the baker, the behavior-shaper; in Schaffner, Cohen, Boston studies in the philosophy of science: PSA 1972 (Reidel, Dordrecht 1974).
Kitchener, R.F.: Behavior and behaviorism. Behaviorism *5:* 11–72 (1977).
Kitchener, R.F.: Piaget's genetic epistemology. Int. Philos. Q. *20:* 377–405 (1980a).
Kitchener, R.F.: Genetic epistemology, normative epistemology and psychologism. Synthese *45:* 257–280 (1980b).
Kitchener, R.F.: The nature and scope of genetic epistemology. Phil. Sci. *48:* 400–415 (1981).
Kitchener, R.F.: Holism and the organismic model in developmental psychology. Hum. Dev. *25:* 233–249 (1982a).
Kitchener, R.F.: Skinner's theory of theories (manuscript submitted for publication, 1982b).
Kitchener, R.F.: Developmental explanations (manuscript submitted for publication, 1982c).
Kitchener, R.F.: Genetic epistemology, history of science and genetic psychology (manuscript submitted for publication, 1982d).
Koch, S.: Psychology and emerging conceptions of knowledge as unitary; in Wann, Behaviorism and phenomenology (University of Chicago Press, Chicago 1964).
Kockelmans, J.J.; Kisiel, T.J.: Phenomenology and the natural sciences (Northwestern University Press, Evanston 1970).
Kuhn, T.: The structure of scientific revolutions (University of Chicago Press, Chicago 1962).
Kuhn, T.: The relations between the history and the philosophy of science; in Kuhn, The essential tension (University of Chicago Press, Chicago 1977).
Kurtines, W.M.: Measurability, description, and explanation: the explanatory adequacy of stage model. Behav. Brain Sci. *2:* 192–194 (1978).
Lakatos, I.: Falsification and the methodology of scientific research programmes; in Lakatos, Musgrave, Criticism and the growth of knowledge (Cambridge University Press, Cambridge 1970).
Lerner, R.M.: Concepts and theories of human development (Addison-Wesley, Reading 1976).
Lerner, R.M.; Skinner, E.A.; Sorell, G.T.: Methodological implications of contextual/dialectic theories of development. Hum. Dev. *23:* 225–235 (1980).
Looft, W.R.: The evolution of developmental psychology. Hum. Dev. *15:* 187–201 (1972).
MacCorquodale, K.; Meehl, P.E.: On a distinction between hypothetical constructs and intervening variables. Psych. Rev. *55:* 95–107 (1948).

Mandelbaum, M.: History, man and reason (Johns Hopkins Press, Baltimore 1971).
Marx, M.: The general nature of theory construction; in Marx, Theories in contemporary psychology (Macmillan, New York 1963).
McCandless, B.R.; Spiker, C.C.: Experimental research in child psychology. Child Dev. 27: 75–80 (1956).
McMullin, E.: The history and philosophy of science: a taxonomy; in Stuewer, Minnesota studies in the philosophy of science, vol. V (University of Minnesota Press, Minneapolis 1970).
McMullin, E.: Structural explanations. Am. Phil. Q. 15: 139–147 (1978).
Mussen, P.H.: Preface; in Mussen, Carmichael's manual of child psychology, vol. I (Wiley, New York 1970).
Nickles, T.: Scientific discovery, logic and rationality (Reidel, Boston 1980a).
Nickles, T.: Scientific discovery: case studies (Reidel, Boston 1980b).
Overton, W.F.: The active organism in structuralism. Hum. Dev. 19: 71–86 (1976).
Overton, W.F.; Reese, W.: Models of development: methodological implications; in Nesselroade, Reese, Life-span developmental psychology: methodological issues (Academic Press, New York 1973).
Pap, A.: Reduction sentences and open concepts. Methods 5: 3–28 (1953).
Piaget, J.: Explanation in psychology and psychophysiological parallelism; in Fraisse, Piaget, Experimental psychology: its scope and method, vol. 1 (Basic Books, New York 1968).
Piaget, J.: Le problème de l'explication; in Apostel et al., L'explication dans les sciences (Flammarion, Paris 1973).
Popper, K.: The logic of scientific discovery; 2nd ed. (Harper & Row, New York 1965).
Radnitzky, G.: Contemporary schools of metascience (Regnery, Chicago 1973).
Rappoport, L.: Naderizing methodology: discussant's comments. Hum. Dev. 23: 218–224 (1980).
Reese, H.W.; Overton, W.F.: Models of development and theories of development; in Goulet, Baltes, Life-span developmental psychology: research and theory (Academic Press, New York 1970).
Reichenbach, H.: Experience and prediction (University of Chicago Press, Chicago 1938).
Rombach, H.: Wissenschaftstheorie (Herder, Freiburg 1974).
Schneewind, K.A.: Wissenschaftstheoretische Grundlagen der Psychologie (Reinhardt, Munich 1977).
Scriven, M.: Explanation and prediction in evolutionary theory. Science 130: 477–482 (1959a).
Scriven, M.: Truisms as the grounds for historical explanations; in Gardiner, Theories of history (Free Press, Glencoe, 1959b).
Seiffert, H.: Einführung in die Wissenschaftstheorie, vol. 2 (Beck, Munich 1978).
Skinner, B.F.: The behavior of organisms (Appleton Century Crofts, New York 1938).
Skinner, B.F.: Current trends in experimental psychology (1947); reprinted in Skinner, Cumulative record; 3rd ed. (Appleton Century Crofts, New York 1972).
Skinner, B.F.: Are theories of learning necessary? (1950); reprinted in Skinner, Cumulative record; 3rd ed. (Appleton Century Crofts, New York 1972).
Stevens, S.S.: Psychology and the science of science. Psych. Bull. 36: 221–263 (1939).
Suppe, F.: The search for philosophical understanding of scientific theories; in Suppe, The structure of scientific theories (University of Illinois Press, Urbana 1974).

Thomas, R.M.: Comparing theories of child development (Wadsworth, Belmont 1979).
Tolman, E.C.: Operational behaviorism and current trends in psychology (1936); reprinted in Tolman, Behavior and psychological man (University of California Press, Berkeley 1951).
Toulmin, S.: Philosophy of science (Harper & Row, New York 1953).
Toulmin, S.: Foresight and understanding (Harper & Row, New York 1961).
Toulmin, S.: Human understanding (Princeton University Press, Princeton 1972).
Turner, M.: Philosophy and the science of behavior (Appleton Century Crofts, New York 1967).
Tweney, R.D.; Doherty, M.E.; Mynatt, C.R.: On scientific thinking (Columbia University Press, New York 1981).
Weimer, W.B.: Notes on the methodology of scientific research (Erlbaum, Hillsdale 1979).
Wolman, B.: Concerning psychology and the philosophy of science; in Wolman, Handbook of general psychology (Prentice-Hall, Englewood Cliffs 1973).
Woodward, J.: Developmental explanations. Synthese *44:* 443–466 (1980).

Beyond Ideology to the Universals of Development

James Youniss[1]

The Catholic University of America, Washington, D.C., USA

In this chapter commentaries are provided on the following topics: (1) the value and shortcomings of critiques of ideology; (2) the misrepresentation of the Piagetian subject as antithetical to critical social theory; (3) the close connections between *Piaget's* thinking and that of one major critical theorist, *Habermas;* (4) the importance of sociological history for developmental psychology, and (5) the need for sociological analysis in appraisal of developmental psychology as a discipline. All of these topics are brought to bear on a single question: What kind of science ought developmental psychology to be? This question is raised in the context of debate regarding the historical choice of positivism as the model of science with which developmental psychology has saddled itself. It is now evident that this model has failed to live up to its promises of keeping knowledge immune from cultural influence and yielding knowledge which is 'objective'. Thus, the discipline faces a new choice of either staying with a model that yields knowledge limited by the constraints of time and place or seeking an alternative that overcomes those limitations and allows the discipline to preserve the goal of knowledge that has universality and generalizability.

The Context

One version of the history of developmental psychology is found in discussions by *Sears* [1975] and *Senn* [1975]. The discipline began in

[1] Work on this chapter was supported in part by a grant from the W.T. Grant Foundation.

the 19th century concerns for child welfare and social reform. Scholars such as *G. Stanley Hall* formed a bridge from philanthropists and moralists to scholars and scientists. As the latter took over these concerns, they sought a foundation in science that would give political action a solid intellectual basis. In the process, the pioneer leaders in the discipline were influenced by experimental psychologists who, themselves, were influenced by physical scientists. The result was adoption of philosophical positivism with its cannons regarding methods for empirical observation and theory construction.

World War Two is a convenient marker for establishing the time when developmental psychology became recognized as a peer among the social sciences. After the war, the discipline was accepted within departments of psychology, and gradually research on development qualified for funding under the rubric of 'basic' science. Subsequently, the discipline experienced expansion in numbers, and from the 1960s on, it gained a new status in society at large. This status included membership in the social-technological elite upon whom government called for expertise in matters of social policy and social problem-solving. For example, establishment of programs such as Head Start was undertaken with consultation from researchers who were called upon to show how research findings could be applied to enhance educational opportunities for children from minority-group backgrounds [*Steiner*, 1976].

While developmental psychology was achieving its present status, the model of science upon which it was consciously built was undergoing dramatic change. *Kuhn* [1962] is often given credit for summarzing many of the weaknesses of positivism, and his book was widely cited across the social sciences. While there appears to have been little debate within developmental psychology regarding positivism, other social sciences, such as sociology, had already uncovered many of positivism's shortcomings [*Berger and Luckmann*, 1967; *Merton*, 1957]. These criticisms opened sociologists to a line of thinking from Europe that was skeptical of positivism and prepared to argue that knowledge had to be looked at according to its origins in historical and social conditions [*Held*, 1980].

'Critical social theory' began to work its way into developmental psychology in the 1970s much through the influence of *Klaus Riegel*. His seminal paper [*Riegel*, 1972] attempted to demonstrate that different types of development theories sprang from discrete national-cultural boundaries. This was to say that psychologists described subjects (children, adolescents, adults) not so much objectively as in terms consonant with historically prevalent ideologies. *Riegel* thus spawned a genre of criticism, taken up in the next section, which accepted the premise that knowledge was a sociological construction and not the product of objective observations synthesized rationally into logical theory.

It is not possible to say precisely where the discipline stands today regarding positivism. Clearly, there is still faith that 'method' is the sure route to truthful knowledge. Yet, there is also increasing awareness that method alone does not guarantee validity or results which are free from limitations of time and place [*Cronbach*, 1975]. One now finds that developmentalists are concerned with temporal specificity of data, as reflected in the concept of 'cohort' [*Elder*, 1980]. And one also finds awareness that theories may be more culture-bound than diligent adherence to methodological tenets would suggest [*Kessen*, 1979; *Sameroff*, 1981].

The once solid front that positivism provided appears to be breaking down. Sufficient skepticism has been voiced to suggest that the discipline is looking for alternatives to the positivistic model. Where it is looking and whether there will be a common focus to its efforts is anything but certain. But it is plausible that in the decade ahead one is likely to see several new models arise, some of which may retain aspects of positivism but most of which are likely to be rather different from it.

Critiques of Ideology

Following *Riegel*, a number of critiques were published, each showing the connection between ideologies in our culture and primary statements in theories. These statements refer to human subjects and imply their 'nature' as well as depict their 'ideal' and most 'advanced' developmental states. Examples include the assumption that subjects are 'self-sufficient individuals' [*Sampson*, 1977] or the proposition that the highest intellectual functioning occurs in 'abstract, formal reasoning' [*Buck-Morss*, 1975]. Statements like the former may be interpreted as expressing the ideology of 'individualism' while the latter may be seen as reflecting a preference for 'mental operations' over 'practical action'.

Although the critiques vary in outlook, they share a common form. A typical critique begins with identification of ideologies that appear to underlie theoretical propositions. It then goes on to explicate the importance of the ideologies in our culture. Next, it makes the point that the propositions found in theories should not be construed as having objectivity. Rather, they are properly understood as having validity for particular social and historical contexts. Finally, it ends with a general statement about critical social theory and the author's intention that the present criticism serve as an occasion for dialogue [*Buck-Morss*, 1975; *Buss*, 1977; *Hogan and Emler*, 1978; *Sampson*, 1977, 1981; *Sullivan*, 1977].

Throughout these critiques, one sees the overall disillusionment with positivism. As a model of science, positivism portrayed scientists as disinterested parties whose adherence to methodological rigor made them immune from personal or social biases. One of the major aims of the critiques is to show that particular methods do not free scientists from these influences. Indeed, by exposing the ideological themes in theories, critics mean to demonstrate that social and historical conditions play a key role in scientists' constructions. The reference to critical social theory serves to advance the argument by suggesting ways in which theory building is a special case of sociological construction, in which prevailing social structures are starting points for scientific thinking. This is to take away any semblance of plausibility to positivism's claim that method is the means by which ideology is superceded and truth is discovered.

It is evident that critiques of ideology have played an important role in the discipline. They have brought debates about positivism into the discipline by applying general arguments to specific developmental theories and concepts. They have also helped introduce developmental psychologists to social constructivism and critical social theory. These are meaningful and timely achievements since they occurred during the 1970s, when the discipline was beginning to express concern over a perceived lack of progress.

Despite these achievements, two questions can be raised concerning this genre of criticism. The first pertains to whether the critiques only enhanced an already smoldering skepticism or whether they provided a way out of this skepticism. The second, and related, issue has to do with the critics' choice of target – *Piaget's* theory.

It is my opinion that the critics have not shown the discipline a credible way of dealing with ideology. On the whole, the critics have used questionable scholarly tactics in rewriting propositions in ideological terms. Following this procedure, anyone is free to nominate any ideology as the correspondent of any proposition [*Broughton*, 1981]. It is no wonder if skepticism is heightened, as nothing is what it says and everything refers ultimately to something else. While the attacks on positivism have clearly served a purpose, the quality of these attacks perhaps does disservice to the theories of focus as well as to promoting insight into critical theory as an antidote to positivism. These points are now pursued in the next two sections, with *Piaget's* theory as the exemplar.

Piaget's Theory

For whatever reason, most of the critiques of ideology in developmental psychology have been centered on structural theories, in particular the theories of *Kohlberg* and *Piaget*. For present purposes, treatment of *Piaget's* theory will be discussed with specific focus on how intellectual development is characterized. Even more arbitrarily, one critique will be considered and treated as representative of the genre. This choice may be unfair to the several arguments that critics have advanced. The only justification offered here is that *Sampson's* [1981] critique is the most recent and, I submit, the most misrepresentative of *Piaget's* position.

Sampson [1981] begins with the assertion that cognitive psychology and, in particular, *Piaget* employ 'an individualistic reduction centered around "I think". Objects are seen to be the products of individual mental operations; the world "out there" is constituted by the individual's thinking and reasoning processes' [*Sampson*, 1981, p. 732]. He elaborates that by giving control to mental operations, theorists cut off operations of thinking subjects 'from their objective roots in social and historical practices' [p. 733]. Further, by placing cognition in individuals' minds, theorists 'cut off people from effective action to change their circumstances rather than their subjective understanding of these circumstances' [p. 733].

Sampson [1981] then depicts *Piaget* as having promoted depiction of 'interaction between active organisms and passive objects' [p. 366]. The consequence is to promote the view of subjects who abhor uncertainty and disorder and who have the capacity to synthesize reality in an orderly fashion. This is done through 'the ability to think abstractly' [p. 736]. It 'involves a purely mental process' of 'decentering' – i.e. 'the ability to get out of one's own shoes, to take on multiple standpoints, and see the world through another's eyes' [p. 736]. In short, *Piaget* is a 'subjectivist' and 'individualist' who grants 'overwhelming primacy to the mental over the material' [p. 737].

Sampson goes on to say that *Piaget* is to be included among those who have committed the error of scientism. *Piaget* has 'adopted one particular interest, the technical, as [the] model for *all* human knowledge' [*Sampson,* 1981, p. 739]. To illustrate, *Sampson* describes *Piaget* as proposing that 'Formal operations represent the highest stage presently known to exist for human cognitive activity' [p. 740]. They are 'the standard of excellence against which all other forms of thinking are judged' [p. 740].

In conclusion, *Sampson* attributes *Piaget's* thinking to several ideologies. They include: 'The demands for technically exploitable, predictable, and controllable knowledge within whose aspect the technical interest constitutes reality' [p. 740]. Or, to 'think abstractly and without interest so that you can better adapt to things as they are; you will be less disturbed than those who insist on frustrating themselves by wanting what they cannot or should not have' [p. 738]. And, *Sampson* presents his own ideological stand in contrast to *Piaget's:* 'The critical study of psychology and society, a study that is self-conscious about its context, its values, and its relationship to human freedom...' [p. 741]; finally, *'to strive toward a psychology not of what is, but of what may yet be'* [p. 742, author's italics].

It is difficult to know where to begin in reacting to *Sampson's* critique. Its semi-accuracy simply destroys any insight *Piaget* tried to provide through his epistemological efforts. The depiction *Sampson* has presented is precisely the one *Piaget* attempted to combat. I take as representative of *Piaget,* and that which separates his work from other contemporary theorists, the following: (1) Knowledge is constituted through interactions between subject and other – either a material object or another subject. (2) The other is not passive but active. The other is *essentially* active and its actions are equal in power to the subject's because they are reciprocal to it. (3) This is why knowledge consists of a subject-other *relation* and not the subject's grasp of the other or the subject's individual construal of the other. (4) Abstraction does not refer to the subject's mental manipulation of other. It is an effort to find regularity in subject-other *interactions* and is inextricably bound to two material end points [*Furth*, 1969; *Youniss*, 1978, 1980]. (5) Decentering is not a mental leap out of self into another's mind. It is to take position different from that with which one has started because subject-other interactions demand such change [*Youniss*, 1981]. (6) Formal operations are results of self-reflections upon concrete operations. They are open to test and revision through hypothetico-deductive reasoning submitted to experimental-empirical testing. (7) As *Sampson* notes, *Piaget* has studied chiefly scientific (mathematical-logical) cognition, but that does not mean that he believed it to be the only type or the standard for all types of knowledge. He distinguished it clearly from knowledge of the social domain [*Piaget*, 1932; *Kitchener*, 1981] and repeatedly referred to *Freud's* work on self-reflection as an important sphere which he had not addressed in his own research.

Sampson and others are free to interpret *Piaget's* writings as they will. However, it is my contention that in taking the tack they have, and thereby ignoring *Piaget's* epistemological uniqueness, they have missed a valuable opportunity to see a theoretical depiction of the intelligent subject that has many of the features that are central to critical theory. By maintaining that *Piaget* has not gone beyond *Kant* and says no more than what other contemporary theorists are saying, the critics have failed to see an insightful revision of classical rationalism that breaks sharply from the positivist model. More unfortunate, they have passed over the opportunity to work constructively with an epistemology that is not alien to critical theory and has proven itself able to generate psychological data. To wit, *Piaget* has tried to demonstrate how persons can be agents responsive to feedback while not replicating it and yet able to transform interactive experience without moving inward to the solopsism of subjective certainty.

Piaget and Habermas

There may be considerably more to share between the epistemological positions of *Piaget* and critical theory than the critics have suggested. Four commonalities are now discussed. Again, a selective choice has been made. For present purposes, critical theory is represented by the writings of and about *Habermas*. Obvious limitations are therefore admitted.

Habermas proposes a three-part division in forms of knowing. The form that most closely corresponds to *Piaget's* work is the *empirical-analytic*. It pertains to humans' *technical* interest and deals with the domain of instrumental actions. For this form, *validity* is constituted in 'hypothetico-deductive theory-testing' in experimentally reproducible conditions. The grounding is in *action* 'involving instrumental feedback-control activity' [*Keat*, 1981, p. 5]. 'Empirical-analytic sciences disclose reality in so far as it appears within the behavioral system of instrumental action ... nomological statements about this object domain ... grasp reality with regard to technical control ...' [*Habermas*, 1971, p. 176].

While the language differs, the elements are similar to *Piaget's*. More important, *Habermas* credits *Piaget* with some epistemological insight that is worth pursuing: 'The stimulus that encouraged me to investigate normative structures from the point of view of developmental logic also came from *Piaget's genetic* structuralism, i.e. from a conception which has overcome the traditional structuralist front against evolutionism and has assimilated motifs of the theory of knowledge from *Kant* to *Peirce*' [*Habermas*, cited in *McCarthy*, 1978, p. 233]. And, 'Following *Piaget*, I suppose that these general structures of cognitive, linguistic, and interactive ability are formed in a simultaneously constructive and adaptive confrontation of the subject with his environment...' [*Habermas*, cited in *McCarthy*, 1978, p. 338].

The *hermeneutic* is a second form of knowledge that refers to interpersonal communication and the domain of symbols. Its validity obtains through consensus in understanding which can be reached between the participants who communicate in a spirit of good will [*Habermas*, 1975, p. 108; *McCarthy*, 1978, p. 288 ff]. *Habermas* recognizes that not all communication can or will lead to consensus. He notes at least four impediments, one of which occurs when one of the participants judges the other not to have rights to perform speech acts. In general, to achieve consensus a 'common definition of the situation is presupposed' or 'is in the process of being worked out' [*McCarthy*, 1978, p. 290].

This brief sketch closely matches *Piaget's* [1932] account of validity in the social-developmental domain. Here, he argued that validity does not obtain in the subject's turning inward to a logical base but in the subject's turning to communication with another in the hope of achieving mutual understanding. The presupposition is that the communicating parties are *equals* who are willing to co-construct valid concepts through mutual accommodation [*Piaget*, 1932, pp. 95, 96; *Kitchener*, 1981; *Youniss*, 1980]. That is, consensus requires use of 'the norm of reciprocity and objective discussion' [*Piaget*, 1932, p. 96]. An impediment to communication occurs in *unilateral* relations when one party takes precedence over the other, blocking off or coercing the other's unput. This impediment corresponds to one described by *Habermas* and permeates *Piaget's* entire discussion of the social domain [*Youniss*, 1978, 1981].

Although this aspect of *Piaget's* work is rarely cited, it is a persistent theme [*Kitchener*, 1981] that is fully compatible with his general epistemology. It should put to rest the conventional interpretation of decentration and role-taking that is falsely attributed to *Piaget*. One person does not come to understand another by mentally imagining what it might be like to be in the other's shoes. Rather, common perspectives are co-constructed through *discussion, debate, argument, negotiation*, and *compromise* [*Piaget*, 1932]. Again, the prerequisite is that the participants seek consensus as equals. That is, they must be operating from a potentially shared definition or seek to construct one together.

A third form of knowledge is *self-reflective*. Its inherent interest is in *emancipation* or *freedom from distortion* [*Keat*, 1981, p. 6]. Validity obtains through success in avoiding self-embedding deception. Validity is achieved through criticism that aids the subject in uncovering biases. While individuals may carry out this process on their own, validity is abetted by the communication process, which involves other persons. As *Keat* [1981] sees the point, communication gives precedence to the hermeneutic form, which spills over and becomes essential to the self-reflective form. Still, for *Habermas* self-reflection is critical since it is essential to the individual's freedom. It can overcome self-deception and stand against authority, so that ultimately the individual can achieve autonomy.

One might see the whole of *Piaget's* corpus as a testament to a similar position. The child's self-reflection requires the actions of objects and other persons. Yet, it does not model them, nor does the child construe them subjectively. More specifically, according to *Piaget* [1932] the communication process is brought in to free the individual from dogmatic authority and to liberate the individual from self-distortion. What then is autonomy? 'Now apart from our relations to other people, there can be no moral necessity. The individual as such knows only anomy... Autonomy therefore appears only with reciprocity, when mutual respect is strong enough to make the individual feel from within the desire to treat others as he himself would wish to be treated' [*Piaget*, 1932, p. 196].

A fourth and important commonality between *Habermas* and *Piaget* is a concern for the *normative* aspects of cognition. Having grounded cognition in action and situating subjects in communicative relations, how can these theorists avoid social-historical reduction so that knowledge deals only in relative truth? One of their answers refers to the *uniformity of process* by which experience of whatever sort is explored for validity. For *Habermas*, emphasis is given to argumentation and discourse to which various claims are submitted [*McCarthy*, 1978, pp. 293 ff.]. Experience, of course, is relative, so truth cannot ensue from correspondence of statement to empirical fact. Rather, 'The condition of the truth of statements is the potential agreement of all others' [*Habermas*, cited in *McCarthy*, 1978, p. 299].

The key idea is that of *intersubjectivity* which refers to a 'procedural realization of universalizability' [*McCarthy*, 1978, p. 314]. In this, *Piaget* is in substantial agreement. For him, cognition of the social domain is not arbitrary or relative when it is grounded in reciprocal discussion between equals. Stress is on the rules of discussion, which dictate that all should be allowed to speak, to be heard, and to work toward mutual understanding [*Piaget*, 1932]. Through this process, individual experience is *transformed*, the result being not endorsement of experience but a normative comprehension of it that, perhaps, neither party initially envisioned but to which both parties can give their assent.

Emphasis on process also holds for the empirical-analytic domain. Here *Habermas* apparently reverts to the ultimate criterion of 'discursive testing'. *Piaget* is more liberal in this regard. Obviously not disregarding this criterion, he also poses the broader notion of *equilibration* as a means to resolve conflicting experiences. Again, the process is one of transforming experience, going beyond it and finding a normative result. *Habermas* recognizes what *Piaget* has attempted: 'The universality of the reference systems within which we objectify reality arises from the development of cognitive operations related to the manipulation of physical objects (things and events). The child learns the logic of using denotative expressions through concrete operations ... and not immediately with grammatical functions' [*Habermas*, cited in *McCarthy*, 1978, pp. 297, 298].

A Need for Revision

I apologize for the use of direct quotations but it was necessary given the degree to which critics have distanced the two positions. I also apologize for what must be seen as a rather superficial treatment of these two theorists. Both are exceedingly complex thinkers in the good sense of the term. *Habermas* has written with a multiple focus on the findings as well as the history of social science. For each answer he achieves, he raises still another question, with an obvious goal of being responsive to philosophically sophisticated discourse, including contemporary debates. *Piaget* is also oriented to philosophical history, as well as contemporary issues in science and philosophy of science.

In describing similarities, I do not mean to say that *Piaget* is a critical theorist or that *Habermas* is a Piagetian. Rather, the point is that they do not differ in the way critics have said or implied. Three general issues should be taken into account. One has to do with their view of the knowing subject. Contrary to the critics' contention, *Piaget* has not formulated an alienated subject who deals in idealized abstractions or seeks subjective self-consistency. His subject is grounded in action, more properly interactions, with regard to material objects and other persons. His is fully a subject of praxis, as is *Habermas's*. It is simply not the case that Piagetian subjects cannot work their way back from thought to material action. Equally important, subjects who are capable of abstract thought have freedom to choose the paths to material action.

A second pertains to the theorist, the scientist or scholar whose task is to study knowledge. It is significant that both *Piaget* and *Habermas* are epistemologists and scientists. They consciously have not operated solely through self-reflection or library research. Rather, they have exposed their thinking to the critical outsider of empirical data. Neither has adopted the model of the theorist as isolated or self-sufficient. Both also recognize the essentialness of remaining in discourse with others, contemporaries as well as historical figures. While this posture has not served *Piaget* well among some psychologists who see no value in *Piaget's* rationale for asking particular questions, the orientation allows others to see him functioning within a tradition compatible with critical theory.

A third general point pertains to their joint concern for *freedom*.

Both assiduously guard the subject's right to generate knowledge through *self-reflection*. They do this necessarily in complex ways in order to preserve other principles such as the possibility of achievement of truth. They avoid making self-reflection subjective license and reject the argument that validity lies merely in self-consistency, self-congruence, or self-satisfaction. They also try to avoid the position that knowledge, grounded in action, is merely relatively true, only to be altered by subsequent experience.

Their emphasis on consensus achieved through argument is recognized as opening the door to other risks. Among these, both have dealt with the problem of authority and coercion, which is a possibility whenever a subject looks to others in the justification process. While there are differences in their respective treatments, the common bond is a denial of consensus through imposition and the demand that, at any moment, all parties have the right to ask for a resumption of discourse in the common search for truth. Despite the fundamentalness of intersubjectivity, self-reflection remains the ultimate act by which individuals retain and justify their freedom.

It is, I think, unfortunate that critics have taken the one clear case in developmental psychology, *Piaget's* theory, as their point of attack and their means of argument against positivism. That model of science seems to be waning of its own accord and, at least, no longer has a strangle-hold over the entire discipline of psychology. *Piaget* is hardly an example of the positivist, nor is his knowing subject its modal characterization. By reframing *Piaget* into an attackable stereotype, the critics have missed a valuable opportunity to help in rebuilding a developmental psychology that is caught already in the trap of relativism and needs a new epistemology to free itself.

Piaget's critics have missed a second opportunity relating to the advancement of critical theory both as a theory for scientific activity and as an epistemological position. To the best of my reading, critical theorists have no theory of psychological development other than a reconstruction of Freudian ideas [*Held,* 1980]. In rereading the critiques of ideology, I found no consistent position on what a developmental theory would look like after *Piaget* was discarded. I do not know whether a full synthesis between Piagetian and critical theory is possible or what the problems are in a merger. However, the initial evidence seems to be sufficiently clear as to warrant initiation of a discussion between the two theories.

Social History

It is possible that some of the critics do not realize or care to face the symbolic meaning which critical theory connotes among social scientists [*Held,* 1980; *Keat,* 1981; *van den Berg,* 1980]. The pioneers in this position were prophets in recognizing positivism's weaknesses and the ills of its offshoot, such as scientism. But they also have been involved in a variety of causes, including justification of anti-intellectual scholarship. Whatever its intent, it should be realized that critical social theory is viewed with caution and wariness for good reason. Perhaps social scientists are just fundamentally conservative and politically naive. But before indicting the lot of us, critics might at least consider that some are open to dialogue when the prospective outcome seems constructive.

In this regard, the specific lines of discourse laid out by critics are hardly inviting. Let me offer a personal interpretation. They would have us discuss propositions about development, and the subject who develops, as concoctions of theorists invested in or simply enculturated to think in terms of capitalism, industrialization, rationalism, technology, and individualism. These, we are told, are the bases of our thinking, since they are the uninspected suppositions from which theories are launched. In not realizing this, we perpetuate the existing social system by legitimizing it in our theories. In the process, we do nothing to change the system or give others cause for altering it. In sum, then, something of a thorough reprogramming is called for, beginning with an expansion of domains and including extension to political action.

Let us focus on only a single element, the investment or enculturation of theorists. What are the constitutive elements of the culture in which we are steeped? How can we know them? In nominating capitalism, industrial forms of production, and the like, critics provide a poor example of the task they lay before psychologists. These abstractions and catch-terms are too general and too vague to be grounds for scholarly debate. To what avail is the reasoning that capitalism implies competition, competition implies individualism, ergo, psychologists begin with the assumption that they must describe the development of individualism, i.e. competence, autonomy, or stablity of personality?

Once the general framework of social construction is accepted, the critics' rationale becomes immediately significant. But that does not, in itself, make their particular analyses useful. Two key steps are missing. The first is an explication of social structure (forces, conditions) that is sociologically credible insofar as it leads to understanding of process. The second is an elaboration that provides historically credible accounts of these processes over time, leading up to present conditions. Mere nomination of ideologies is no substitute for this program. Capitalism, as a chief example, has been with us for over 500 years, so to say that it underlies psychological theories is equivalent to saying not much of anything. I, for one, would not become critical of a science that failed to calculate 'capitalism' into the picture.

It is fortuitous for developmental psychologists interested in this type of project that the kind of analysis needed is already underway. The largest body of work appears in the discipline of social history, which combines historical study with demography, economics, politics, and sociology. Developmentalists were introduced to this discipline through *Aries'* [1962] study, which is frequently cited in elementary texts. While some of the citations present the study as showing how society thought of childhood before developmental scientists discovered its true significance, the work goes well beyond 'pre-scientific' description. As the subtitle indicates, this *Social Historical Study of Family Life* attempted to identify social structural changes that led to alterations of family life by reordering relations among members as well as between members and society at large.

Aries' [1962] study opened a floodgate of research from which results are still pouring out in a torrent. Recent summaries of this research show its breadth as well as indicate the complexity involved in finding consensus explanations [*Stone,* 1981]. One point on which there is agreement, however, is that the family as we know it today is not a product of modernization, which in the USA refers to phenomena occurring roughly from 1850 up to the present. The nuclear family consisting of a couple, separated from their families of origin, plus their offspring did not emerge with capitalism or industrialization. It arose earlier. This is true, in part, if only because demographics did not permit extended families; indeed, they rarely allowed parents to live long enough to be witnesses at all their children's weddings [*Fischer,* 1978; *Glick and Parke,* 1965].

Family social history has been closely allied with studies of segmented aspects of the life cycle: childhood [*Greven,* 1977], youth [*Gillis,* 1974; *Kett,* 1977], and old age [*Fischer,* 1978]. These studies, in turn, are coupled with research on women [*Bernard*, 1981; *Branca*, 1978; *Degler*, 1980], on education [*Tyack*, 1974], and work [*Sennet*, 1974]. What one finds in all of this work is a tightly interwoven, but as yet not well-understood, set of conditions that have realigned roles for individuals and rearranged relations among them. A comparison of *Degler* [1980] and *Kett* [1977] provides an interesting case that is germaine to contemporary developmental psychology.

The importance of motherhood to children's development is uncontestably central to many developmental theories. *Degler* [1980] has attempted to document how the motherhood role became structured and how its significance evolved. He hypothesizes that the restructuring occurred in the USA around 1780–1820, when wage-earning drew men cut of the house and business practices imposed new rules of conduct on them. This resulted in a *separation of spheres* and led to a sharp division between men's and women's domains. It also gave women a singular presence in the home and helped to invest them with authority over children. The process further abetted the perception of women as preservers of morality, in part as a contrast to rules of conduct in the outside world.

Kett's [1977] complementary work helps to show how motherhood became the superordinate concept with respect to childhood. Among other things, childhood took on a new significance especially with regard to moral training. In one of the more interesting, but not obvious, derivatives, *Kett* points out that later in the 19th century, men re-entered children's lives, specifically, when children became youth. One of their tasks was to reorient youth to the man's world via character toughening, which *Kett* calls 'muscular Christianity'. This movement took on added import as employment opportunities for boys waned, leaving them with physical energy but few productive outlets. Among the responses was the high school.

This sketch provides an illustration of what is meant by social historical analysis that deals in *process* explanation. A restructuring here is followed by a response there, and so on, as a chain evolves. The argument is not that we know all the links. Rather, it is that social historians have gone much farther in seeking a social analysis than psychologists have done or can do on their own. That this is a productive line to pursue is evident from the work of *Gadlin* [1977, 1978a, b]. He has used the interdisciplinary process analysis to evaluate concepts that recur throughout contemporary psychological theory. *Gadlin's* work represents hermeneutical research that bears on theories of husband-wife relations, child-rearing practices, and self-concept development.

A second line of research appears in societal analysis contained more within sociology proper. Two authors of obvious interest to developmentalists are *Riesman* [1950] and *Bell* [1973]. Both present process accounts that are framed with historical sensitivity. *Riesman's* study unfortunately has not been accorded the place it might have in developmental theories dealing with child-rearing. Such theories, as is well-known, typically begin with observations of rearing practices; these observations are then categorized and correlated with behavioral outcomes in children. Few researchers have asked why parents use different practices in the first place or whether the observed outcomes might not arise as well from factors other than the child-rearing practices.

Riesman [1950] identified three general types of character that correspond to three broad historical eras. These eras refer to discrete kinds of social organization, each dominated by a peculiar set of rules covering interpersonal relations. According to *Riesman*, in an *inner-directed* world, the belief was that a person's stable character, or lack of it, was responsible for social success or failure. Parents operating from this belief were responsible when they attempted to cultivate aspects of character necessary for success. By contrast, in an *outer-directed* world, stable traits are of lesser value. The more successful mode puts the premium on adaptability and flexibility to changing circumstances. Among other things, when change is the rule, parents cannot know which traits to foster, other than those that underlie the readiness to readapt. These two eras require distinct types of child-rearing. And the latter includes the real possibility that parents will voluntarily recede to the background, letting peers, teachers, and others determine where and how socialization should proceed.

Another, briefer illustration is provided by *Bell* [1973], who analyzes society's reorganization from the pre-industrial through the present 'post-industrial' period. He also uses the process approach, such as in describing social class: 'Class, in the final sense, denotes not a specific group of persons but a system that has institutionalized the ground rules for acquiring, holding, and transferring differential power and its attendant privileges' [*Bell*, 1973, p. 361]. It is worth noting that *Bell's* depiction of post-industrial society assigns prestige, power, and control to those who possess technical knowledge and skill, who have acquired current methods through advanced education, and who operate as individuals seeking a better future, rather than to persons seeking to perpetuate property, traditional values, or family background. One cannot help but see in this analysis a more solid sociological ground to serve as a foundation for contemporary theories of cognition. The mind modeled after the computer, the mentality which manages information through self-control processing strategies, fulfills the prerequisites of the power elite in post-industrial society.

The third, and least developed, line of research is that in which scientific disciplines are studied as *institutions*. Institutional structures and dynamics are considered as parts of the process by which knowledge is engendered. This subfield has been called the *sociology of knowledge* [*Merton*, 1957, chapter XII] and has not evolved very far in the case of developmental psychology. What has been written appears aimed at getting developmentalists interested in studying their own discipline's institutional structure [*Donzelot*, 1979; *Lasch*, 1980; *McCarthy*, 1981; *Steiner*, 1976].

Several hypotheses have guided work so far. One of these is that the rise of modern states has become associated with efforts to control ever more segments of peoples lives [*Boli-Bennett and Meyer*, 1978]. Childhood is an especially opportune candidate in that efforts at regulation can be justified in terms of potential benefits. For example, medical care and education may be seen as goods and eventually as necessities or rights, so that questions about control are eclipsed [*Steiner*, 1976]. Gradually, the issue of regulation enters into matters of law and can result in disputes between parents and the state as to which has responsibility for children's care and regulation of their behavior [*Burt*, 1980]. From this perspective, a set of tightly aggregated presuppositions have come to be associated with childhood in the modern era. The set has been established through the creation of institutions, laws, and expectations cast as duties and rights.

Kessen [1979] and *Skolnick* [1975], among contemporary developmentalists, seem sensitive to this line of reasoning. They have been willing to raise the question of whether our formal theories of childhood are as much due to scientific discovery as they are to *invention* of the culture of which developmentalists are a part. *Platt* [1969], in a study of the 'child saving' movement and treatment of delinquency of the late 19th century, has raised this same question in a provocative way. He notes that propositions about child-rearing and early experiences in the family came into public view long before there was scientific evidence on their behalf. These propositions now appear in scientific theories substantially unchanged but with the stamp of evidence that gives them legitimacy in a technological sense.

An open-mindedness to this position raises the question of whether developmental psychologists are the movers behind ideas or simply moved by the culture to adopt ideas [*Kessen,* 1979]. The notion of state control surely complicates the question, given that some developmentalists have sought to apply their theories in the service of the public good. They have offered their theories by way of expert testimony in matters of policy-making, legal decisions, and legislation and, in so doing, have enhanced state control. In a more subtle version of the same point, psychologists' appeal to public funds for university education and research may produce the same result. Only recently have psychologists begun to inspect this relation and to probe its broader implications [*Bevan,* 1980].

A second hypothesis also deals with power but concentrates on the role of professionals in technologically oriented cultures. One of the dramatic sectors of growth during this century has been in employment categories that offer human services [*Bell,* 1973]. While developmentalists tend to think of themselves not as professionals but as researchers and scholars, the content of their work and its implications put them in association with what *Donzelot* [1979] has coined 'the *psy* professions'. *Lasch* [1979, 1980] has viewed these professions, in part, as helping to create the 'therapeutic state' and, in part, as maintaining themselves through self-interest. In the latter vein, professions compete for power by making their knowledge essential or critical. They do this by creating problems for which only they can claim technical solutions.

According to either of these hypotheses, developmental psychology is characterized as caught in strong historical trends which have given it a definite role to play. This view dashes the old image of the isolated scholar who makes quiet discoveries in the laboratory. The new image reflects a recognition that science is a public enterprise that is not isolated from society but is very much a part of and responsive to it. As this image seeps into the discipline, it may provoke its members to look more carefully at what they do, not in terms of methodological purity so much as from the perspective of cultural analysis.

What seems to be called for is a deeper concern for history. Only recently have developmentalists begun to explore this topic [*Sears,* 1975; *Senn,* 1975]. However, neither *Sears* nor *Senn* get far enough into sociological history to address the questions raised above. It is interesting to note that much of the work cited here, including the critiques of ideology, constitute a revisionistic account of the discipline, what it has done, and why it has done it. In the absence of developmentalists' interest in analyzing their discipline, it may be that revisions will appear before the original history is written.

Conclusion

The single most important issue facing developmental psychology stems from the demise of positivism that is still in process. As developmentalists become aware that they can no longer rely on this model of science, they face a dilemma. If they concentrate on methods of data collection and analysis, they can gain assurance that what they find is verifiable, but at the cost of loss of generality [*Cronbach*, 1975]. Psychologists then become chroniclers of the present but give up the vision of seeking the general, the universal, and the lawful [*Edelstein*, 1981]. The alternative is not to give up this ethos that has driven social scientists for the past several hundred years [*Becker*, 1967]. To take this road, however, developmentalists have to start from a different definition of science and perhaps create that science anew.

What kind of science ought developmental psychology to be? Following from the arguments that have been presented here, two of its key components would be sociology and sociological history. They seem essential both for self-understanding of the discipline and for appropriate conceptualization of the individuals who are the subjects of our studies. Earlier in this century, developmental psychology consciously affiliated with the parent discipline of experimental psychology with the clear objective of becoming scientific. It is now widely recognized as having achieved that status, but at considerable cost. What is not recognized is that in adopting positivism, developmentalists severed themselves from intellectual traditions that offer insights that cannot be achieved from online observation of here-and-now behavior.

This paper began with a discussion of critiques of ideology as they have been applied to structural theories. It was argued that these critiques offer insufficient reason to abandon those theories. It was argued that *Piaget's* theory, in particular, provides an epistemology that goes beyond positivism and makes essential connections with critical social theory. I have liberalized the definition of critical theory for the sake of illustrating the value of thinking of knowledge as the product of social construction. When applied to developmental psychology, analysis in terms of social construction places the discipline in a historical and sociological context and, by necessity, does the same for the subjects of our studies.

The goal is to move beyond positivism, which has encouraged us to follow stilted methods with the promise of truth as the outcome. It has, instead, dimmed our self-consciousness and produced results restricted to accounts limited by time and place. A developmental psychology without generalized laws and universal processes is not a science in the full sense. A model of social construction offers no guarantee and, surely, also can result in knowledge that is relative. But it need not, and representatives of it, such as *Piaget* and *Habermas,* have not lost the vision that the discipline needs. Developmentalists do not have to give up the concern for methodology that positivism engendered. Indeed, they should not. But method alone is not the answer. It should be supplemented with sociology and sociological history. Therein lies the makings of science that can deal with ideology and get beyond it.

Summary

Critics of the discipline of developmental psychology have made a broadside attack, challenging its model of science as well as its ideological implications. Some of their arguments are plausible but the whole is confusing and leads in too many directions at once. It is suggested that the future science of development can rectify past errors and maintain its original vision through two major steps. One is to adopt an epistemology of social construction and the other is to form a serious scholarly alliance with sociology and social history. Review of findings from these disciplines is offered to show how concepts of development may be clarified when the organism as well as the theorist are set in a definite historical-social context.

References

Aries, P.: Centuries of childhood: A social history of family life (Knopf, New York 1962).
Becker, E.: The structure of evil (Free Press, New York 1967).
Bell, D.: The coming of post-industrial society (Basic Books, New York 1973).
Berg, A. van den: Critical theory: Is there still hope? Am. J. Sociol. 86: 449–478 (1980).

Berger, P.L.; Luckmann, T.: The social construction of reality (Doubleday, Garden City 1967).
Bernard, J.: The female world (Free Press, New York 1981).
Bevan, W.: On getting in bed with a lion. Am. Psychol. *35:* 779–789 (1980).
Boli-Bennett, J.; Meyer, J.W.: The ideology of childhood and the state. Am. sociol. Rev. *43:* 797–812 (1978).
Branca, P.: Women in Europe since 1750 (St. Martin's Press, New York 1978).
Broughton, J.M.: Piaget's structural developmental psychology. V. Ideology-critique and the possibility of a critical developmental theory. Hum. Dev. *24:* 382–411 (1981).
Buck-Morss, S.: Socio-economic bias in Piaget's theory and its implications for cross-cultural studies. Hum. Dev. *18:* 35–49 (1975).
Burt, R.A.: The constitution of the family; in Kurland, Casper, The Supreme Court Review, 1979. (University of Chicago Press, Chicago 1980).
Buss, A.R.: The emerging field of the sociology of psychological knowledge. Am. Psychol. *30:* 988–1002 (1975).
Buss, A.R.: Piaget, Marx, and Buck-Morss on cognitive development. Hum. Dev. *20:* 118–128 (1977).
Cronbach, L.J.: Beyond the two disciplines of scientific psychology. Am. Psychol. *30:* 116–127 (1975).
Degler, C.: At odds: women and the family in America from the revolution to the present (Oxford University Press, New York 1980).
Donzelot, J.: The policing of families (Pantheon, New York 1979).
Edelstein, W.: Cultural constraints on development and the vicissitudes of progress. Houston Symp. IV on Psychology and Society: The child and other cultural inventions, 1981.
Elder, G.H., Jr.: Adolescence in historical perspective; in Adelson, Handbook of adolescent psychology (Wiley, New York 1980).
Fischer, D.H.: Growing old in America (Oxford University Press, New York 1978).
Furth, H.G.: Piaget and knowledge (Prentice Hall, Englewood Cliffs 1969).
Gadlin, H.: Private lives and public order; in Levinger, Rausch, Close relationships (University of Massachusetts Press, Amherst 1977).
Gadlin, H.: Child discipline and the pursuit of self; in Reese, Lippsitt, Advances in child development and behavior, vol. 13 (Academic Press, New York 1978a).
Gadlin, H.: Scars and emblems: paradoxes of American family life. J. soc. Hist. *11:* 305–327 (1978b).
Gillis, J.R.: Youth and history (Academic Press, New York 1974).
Glick, P.C.; Parke, R.: New approaches in studying the life cycle of the family. Demography *2:* 187–202 (1965).
Greven, P.: The protestant temperament: patterns of child-rearding, religious experience, and the self in early America (New American Library, New York 1977).
Habermas, J.: Knowledge and human interests (Beacon Press, Boston 1971).
Habermas, J.: Legitimation crisis (Beacon Press, Boston 1975).
Held, D.: Introduction to critical theory (University of California Press, Berkeley 1980).
Hogan, R.T.; Emler, N.P.: The biases in contemporary social psychology. Soc. Res. *45:* 478–534 (1978).
Keat, R.: The politics of social theory (University of Chicago Press, Chicago 1981).

Kessen, W.: The American child and other cultural inventions. Am. Psychol. *34:* 815-820 (1979).
Kett, J.: Rites of passage (Basic Books, New York 1977).
Kitchener, R.F.: Piaget's social psychology. J. Theory social Behav. (1981).
Kuhn, T.S.: The structure of scientific revolutions (University of Chicago Press, Chicago 1962).
Lasch, C.: Haven in a heartless world (Basic Books, New York 1979).
Lasch, C.: Life in the therapeutic state. N.Y. Rev. Books *July 12* (1980).
McCarthy, J.: Who wants a national policy on children and families. Social Thought *7:* 9-21 (1981).
McCarthy, T.: The critical theory of Jürgen Habermas (MIT Press, Cambridge 1978).
Merton, R.K.: Social theory and social structure (Free Press, Glencoe 1957).
Piaget, J.: The moral judgment of the child (Routledge Kegan Paul, London 1932).
Platt, A.: The child savers (University of Chicago Press, Chicago 1969).
Riegel, K.F.: The influence of economic and political ideologies on the development of developmental psychology. Psychol. Bull. *78:* 129-141 (1978).
Riegel, K.F.: The dialectics of human development. Am. Psychol. *1976:* 689-700.
Riesman, D.: The lonely crowd: a study of changing American character. (Doubleday, Garden City 1950).
Sameroff, A.J.: Development and the dialectic; in Collins, 15th Minnesota Symp. on Child Psychology (Erlbaum, Hillsdale 1981).
Sampson, E.E.: Psychology and the American ideal. J. Personal. soc. Psychol. *35:* 767-782 (1977).
Sampson, E.E.: Cognitive psychology as ideology. Am. Pschol. *36:* 730-743 (1981).
Sears, R.R.: Your ancients revisited; in Hetherington, Review of child development research (University of Chicago Press, Chicago 1975).
Senn, M.J.E.: Insights on the child development movement in the United States. Monogr. 40, serial No. 161 (Society for Research in Child Development, 1975).
Sennett, R.: Families against the city (Vintage Books, New York 1974).
Skolnick, A.: The limits of childhood: conceptions of child development and social context. Law contemp. Probl. *39:* 38-77 (1975).
Steiner, G.Y.: The children's cause (Brookings Institution, Washington 1976).
Stone, L.: Family history in the 1980s. J. interdiscipl. Hist. *12:* 51-87 (1981).
Sullivan, E.V.: A study of Kohlberg's structural theory of moral development: a critique of liberal social science ideology. Hum. Dev. *20:* 352-376 (1977).
Tyack, D.B.: The one best system (Harvard University Press, Boston 1974).
Youniss, J.: Dialectical theory and Piaget on social knowledge. Hum. Dev. *21:* 234-247 (1978).
Youniss, J.: Parents and peers in social development (University of Chicago Press, Chicago 1980).
Youniss, J.: A revised interpretation of Piaget (1932); in Sigel et al., New directions in Piagetian theory and practice (Erlbaum, Hillsdale 1981).

Developmental Analysis: A Strategy for the Study of Psychological Change

Alexander W. Siegel[a], *Jeffrey Bisanz*[b], *Gay L. Bisanz*[b]

[a] University of Houston, Houston, Tex., USA;
[b] University of Alberta, Edmonton, Alberta, Canada

A major goal of psychology has been to establish a set of procedures and theories to describe, measure, predict, and modify the behavior of organisms. A less emphasized but increasingly important concern is understanding how that behavior changes or develops.

'It is convenient to distinguish between the 'space arts', those in which a glimpse of the world is cast into permanent form in picture, statue, or building, and the 'time arts', those in which the arrangement of words, tones, or bodily movements captures the flowing character of all temporally ordered experience. We may, in a similar fashion, distinguish between the sciences which capture and describe the structured and episodic arrangements of the world of things and events and those which concern themselves with change through time. The life sciences have been rapidly moving from structural-episodic inquiry to temporal-development inquiry' [*Murphy and Kovach*, 1972, p. 399].

'Temporal-development' inquiry requires procedures for the investigation of development. One purpose of this paper is to argue that a partial set of such conceptual and empirical procedures already exists.

Paradoxically, in psychology the term 'development' is used both too narrowly and too widely. Some psychologists consider the process of development to be functionally synonymous with 'child development'. To be sure, 'development' does occur in childhood, but it also occurs in a large number of other biological, psychological, and social contexts. Other psychologists label many kinds of change 'development', whether they are referring to motor development in infancy or developmental processes in aging. Used in both these senses, 'development' is entirely a descriptive, empirical term synonymous with 'change'; nothing in particular is implied about the nature of change beyond its mere occurrence. So defined, the term 'development' is applied to changes that happen to occur within the traditional domains of developmental psychology. Most important, such a definition provides no guidelines for conceptualizing and investigating behavioral change. As a result, *McCandless and Geis* [1975] were able to characterize developmental psychology as a healthy collection of normative and empirical research data, without considering whether researchers share a common agenda of goals and methods that is sufficient to define the field as a distinct subdiscipline. As *White* [1970] has argued so eloquently, a shared agenda is vital to the health of a research community. In our view, developmental psychology is diverging from, rather than converging on, such an agenda.

Our intent is to describe a framework for research and theory that can provide a common agenda for developmental psychologists in diverse areas. Within this framework, not all types of change in the traditional domains of developmental psychology constitute instances of development. Conversely, certain changes that occur in other contexts (e.g. embryogenesis, learning, and personality changes in adults) may constitute instances of development. Defining development in a theoretical and limited sense has historical precedence, although discordant with contemporary practice. We are not wedded to the particular definition of development employed in this chapter. In fact, later we will argue that this definition is too imprecise and must be replaced by a definition based on more specific and theoretically valuable concepts. Our purpose in defining development in this manner is primarily didactic: It allows us to focus selectively on a specific kind of change and on a perspective and general procedures for investigating that change. We will call this framework and approach 'developmental analysis' and try to demonstrate its applicability to problems of change in a variety of psychological contexts.

The characteristics of developmental analysis, as we are defining the term, are not new, nor do they spring forth in whole cloth from any one theory or the work of a single investigator. Rather, they have an extended and often implicit history of partial employment in various disciplines and have been used in achieving a variety of scientific agenda. These characteristics are the core of *Spencer's* [1862, 1864, 1870, 1904] 'development hypothesis', or 'doctrine of evolution', and have been integral to the thinking of every serious developmentalist from *Baldwin* to *Werner* to *Piaget* [*Grinder,* 1968]. Our goal is to delineate a contemporary form of developmental analysis. We view this general approach as providing an organizing framework that developmental psychology currently lacks.

In the first two sections of this paper, we draw examples from historical and contemporary research and theory to instantiate this general perspective on development and the procedures of inquiry generated by it. In the final section, we discuss limitations and potential extensions of the approach as well as the benefits of defining developmental psychology as a set of shared conceptual and empirical methods for studying change.

*Contemporary Developmental Analysis:
The Developmental Perspective*

The general approach of contemporary developmental analysis can be best understood with reference to a long-standing theory of human perception and thought, labeled by *Bergson* [1911] as the 'cinematographical mechanism' [*Blumenthal,* 1977; *Ribot,* 1911; *Siegel,* 1977; *Spencer,* 1862]. From this perspective, the fundamental nature of the world is continuous activity and change [*Riegel,* 1976]. However, this change cannot be perceived directly. While it is *change* that is real, the human knowledge system is predisposed to abstract or hypostatize *states* or 'snapshots'. 'Our mind, which seeks solid bases of operation, has as its principal function ... to imagine *states* and *things*' [*Bergson,* 1922, p. 222]. Change is perceived on the basis of differences between these successively abstracted states.

Developmental analysis involves a strategy very similar to that of the 'cinematographical mechanism'. Like the perceiver of change, the investigator of change cannot observe it directly. 'The problem is to impose order and organization on the activity and thus establish a workable stability, or momentary constancy in the face of change' [*Overton,* 1975, p. 65]. The investigative strategy implied is to conceptualize change as 'temporal events divisible into successive stages' [*Werner,* 1957, p. 128] or states and subsequently to find patterns in the succession of these 'Bergsonian snapshots'. Thus, while the primary focus of developmental analysis is on describing and understanding *change,* in so doing it is necessary to specify the characteristics of the abstracted *states.*

How Are the States Characterized?

Organized Systems. The hypostatized states are not merely collections of independent elements. Rather, each state is viewed as a system whose elements are interrelated and organized; such a system has unique properties distinct from the properties of its constituents [*Piaget,* 1970; *Sutherland,* 1973]. Systems of this type are called (interchangeably) wholes, organizations, or structures.

In psychology, there are numerous conceptualizations in which this notion of an organized system is central. For example, *Bischof* [1975] has proposed a control model of social behavior in which he details various internal and external factors in the development of attachment and fear responses and specifies how they become coordinated. In current models of semantic memory [*Smith,* 1978], it is proposed that the meaning of a specific concept, rather than being represented as a single lexical entry, is derived from various relational links with other concepts. In these examples, as in developmental analysis, structure is not simply a convenient construct to be explained eventually by a more detailed analysis of the isolated constituents. Rather, structure per se (i.e. the organizational relationships) is an essential part of the explanation [*Overton,* 1975].

Hierarchical Organization. Any organized system is both a superordinate organization of its own constituents (as described above) and simultaneously a subordinate constituent in a higher-level system. In other words,

> 'What (are) wholes on one level (are) parts on a higher one. Each level of organization possesses unique properties of structures and behavior which, though dependent on the properties of the constituent elements, appear only when these elements are combined in the new system. Knowledge of the laws of the lower level is necessary for a full understanding of the higher level; yet the unique properties of phenomena at the higher level cannot be predicted, a priori, from the laws of the lower level' [*Novikoff,* 1945, p. 209].

Multi-level systems of this type are referred to as *hierarchically organized* systems. Within this context, 'hierarchy' refers to an organization in which the activities of a lower level are integrated and represented at a higher level. It does not refer to a linear ordering along a single dimension, such as *Hull's* [1943] 'habit-family hierarchy' (which is ordered in terms of response strength).

The principle of hierarchical organization is exemplified in *Jackson's* [1884] extension of *Spencer's* development hypothesis to the evolution, structure, and function of the nervous system. According to the Jacksonian view, evolution (development) is characterized as a progression from simplicity and automaticity toward greater complexity, flexibility, and voluntary control. The central nervous system is organized as a set of centers or levels of integration, each center being more evolved and developed (i.e. more complex, flexible, and less automatic) than the centers immediately below it. The lower centers 'represent' most simply and directly sensory and motor information concerning movement from a given portion of the body. Movement information from a number of lower centers is 're-represented' in a more complex fashion at the level of the middle centers; similarly, information from the middle centers is 're-re-represented' at the level of the higher centers. The higher centers coordinate the activity of subordinate centers, are the last to evolve completely, involve the greatest complexity, and are most subject to voluntary control.

Jackson [1874] hypothesized that certain disease processes act upon higher centers, disrupting the flow of information between higher and lower centers and, specifically, diminishing the control of higher over lower centers. Behavioral manifestations of the disorder (e.g. hallucinations, bizarre and uncontrolled gestures) were interpreted as being due to the action of the *highest remaining intact center,* now lacking the control typically exercised by its dysfunctional superordinate center. Using this model of the nervous system, *Jackson* and his successors were able to make important strides in understanding epilepsy, hemiplegia, chorea, and, more generally, brain-behavior relationships. The principle of hierarchical organization continues to have important implications for the contemporary study of brain evolution [*Jerison,* 1976; *MacLean,* 1970; *Rozin,* 1976], developmental neurology [*Milner,* 1967], contemporary theoretical biology [*Bertalanffy,* 1967, 1968; *Pattee,* 1973], and cognitive development [*Fischer,* 1980; *Piaget,* 1971; *Siegel* et al., 1978].

The concept of hierarchical organization represents a specific solution to the problem of how an organism continually adapts while at the same time maintaining its functional integrity in the face of change. As a higher level is being constructed, or in the event that a higher level fails (as in 'regression' or in psychopathology), the lower level remains operative, so that the function in question is preserved. A related property of hierarchically organized systems concerns the *rate* at which complex systems might evolve. *Simon* [1973, pp. 7, 8] has illustrated this property with a parable:

'Two watchmakers assemble fine watches, each watch containing ten thousand parts. Each watchmaker is interrupted frequently to answer the phone. The first has organized his total assembly operation into a sequence of subassemblies; each subassembly is a stable arrangement of 100 elements, and each watch, a stable arrangement of 100 subassemblies. The second watchmaker has developed no such organization. The average interval between phone interruptions is a time long enough to assemble about 150 elements. An interruption causes any set of elements that does not yet form a stable system to fall apart completely. By the time he has answered about eleven phone calls, the first watchmaker will usually have finished assembling a watch. The second watchmaker will almost never succeed in assembling one – he will suffer the fate of Sisyphus: As often as he rolls the rock up the hill, it will roll down again.'

The principle of hierarchical organization may well be an important key to understanding the rapid changes that occur in the course of development.

How Is Development Characterized?

Invariant Sequence. Given the infinite number of phenomena in which change may be observed, the investigator must focus on instances that have considerable generality. If outcomes X, Y, and Z are observed to occur in any order (like the child's acquisition of the verbs 'run', 'catch', and 'see'), there is no reason to suspect that the three are related to each other in a manner that is essential to understanding the successive changes. The order of succession for each case (i.e. each child) is likely to be regulated by some random or ungeneralizable process. However, if X, Y, and Z always occur in a unique order, i.e. in an *invariant sequence,* then it is likely that the progression is regulated by a process that is consistent and generalizable across individuals. For example, *Gentner* [1975] has shown that children's acquisition of the verbs 'give', 'trade', and 'sell' occurs in a unique order. According to her analysis of possession verbs, this sequence can be accounted for by the ordered acquisition of semantic components and relations, the meaning of verbs acquired earlier being embedded in the meanings of verbs acquired later. Thus, an invariant sequence provides a clue to understanding the processes controlling the sequence.

Invariant sequences are recurrent regularities that are central to developmental analysis. Discovery of such sequences raises the possibility that the successive structures underlying change may be characterized by certain principles or mechanisms and that the procedures of developmental analysis (to be described later) can be applied heuristically to understand the change involved. Thus, a necessary condition for any developmental theory is the existence of sequential regularity in behavioral change. An invariant sequence represents a particularly interesting regularity that, like other regularities in nature, serves as a focal point for scientific investigation.

Definition. In developmental analysis the focus is on a particular type of invariant sequence: 'Development' is defined as change in the direction of increasing differentiation and hierarchic integration [*Kaplan,* 1966, 1967; *Piaget,* 1971; *Spencer,* 1864; *Werner,* 1948]. In this context, *differentiation* is the process by which the components of a 'whole' become distinguished from each other; the 'whole' may be any structure, such as a physical entity, a motor routine, a schema, or a mental process. *Hierarchic integration* is the process by which these components become related to one another in a hierarchical organization. The operation of these two complementary processes is exemplified in embryological development. An embryo begins as a single cell, but it divides rapidly into distinct cells that form specific body tissues. These new tissues are not independent; rather, they are integrated into the muscular, respiratory, digestive, and other systems. These systems, in turn, are coordinated in a plan for overall body functioning.

The same process occurs in behavioral development, although the components and their organization may be less directly observable. For example, in the acquisition of fine motor skills (such as playing a musical instrument), individual movements become distinct from each other while simultaneously becoming coordinated into a goal-oriented, patterned system of action. In semantic development, concepts like 'apple' and 'orange' or 'mitosis' and 'meiosis' not only become more distinct in meaning, but they also become integrated into superordinate conceptual categories such as 'fruit' or 'cell division'. In these examples and in development generally, the two processes are reciprocal, with integration guiding the way in which components are differentiated, and differentiation influencing the nature of integration.

Using this limited definition, many kinds of change often described as being 'developmental' are not the focus of developmental analysis. Thus, simple changes in height and weight are nondevelopmental, as are the multiplication of cancer cells, and the unstructured sprawl of suburbs. An increase with age in memory span is considered developmental if, and only if, it is construed as an outcome of underlying changes characterized by increasing differentiation and integration (e.g., chunking operations). The same can be said of simple substitutions in, or additions to, a cognitive repertoire [*Flavell*, 1972].

These cases serve to illustrate the point that the term 'development', as used here, is strictly a theoretical concept. *Werner and Kaplan* [1956] referred to this definition as the 'orthogenetic principle' and described its use to investigators as follows: 'This principle has the status of heuristic "law". Though not itself subject to empirical test, it is valuable to developmental psychologists in directing inquiry and in determining the actual range of applicability with regard to the behavior of organisms' [*Werner and Kaplan*, 1956, p. 866]. Obviously, this definition must be evaluated according to its heuristic value for research and theory; later we return to this issue. The point to emphasize, however, is that developmental analysis is concerned with identifying theoretical classes of change that focus and direct inquiry.

The Role of Time. Although developmental change occurs over time (or age), time itself causes nothing [*Kaplan*, 1967; *Spiker*, 1966; *Werner and Kaplan*, 1956; *Wohlwill*, 1970]. In developmental analysis, temporal variables such as time and age serve the function of a 'stalking horse'. That is, time and age are used initially as consensual indices or markers to study the development of a system. But once an invariant sequence of states has been represented, the temporal indices are of less consequence [*Siegel and White*, 1975]. What remains is an ordered sequence of state-representations that can be used to make inferences about the nature of change in the system. *Kohlberg* [1963], for example, used age initially as a convenient index to distinguish successive levels (states) of moral reasoning. Once 'age-related' states were specified, ordered, and confirmed to *Kohlberg's* satisfaction, age became irrelevant. What remained were six distinct modes of moral reasoning, ordered in terms of progressive complexity. Though there remains a significant dispute about the sequential invariance and accuracy of *Kohlberg's* stages of moral reasoning [*Kurtines and Grief*, 1974], the value of the general approach lies in what can be learned about *sequences* of behavioral development. The emphasis is on what occurs and how it comes about, not on when.

Given that time and age may become 'throw-away' variables, it is clear that the spans of time over which development is studied are arbitrary in theory (though not necessarily in practice). Developmental analysis may be applied to sequences of states that occur over diverse temporal spans, depending on the nature of the problem and the purpose of the investigator [*White and Siegel,* 1976]. Thus, in looking at changes in system characteristics, states may be constructed to represent organizations over temporal durations as varied as milliseconds (as in the microgenesis of perception), seconds and minutes (as in problem-solving), months and years (as in the ontogenesis of thought, language, and socialization), or even millions of years (as in phylogenesis).

Contemporary Developmental Analysis: Procedures of Inquiry

How might effective procedures for research be derived from this theoretical perspective? The details of any particular inquiry will, of course, depend on the problem domain and the research tools available (e.g. statistical techniques, experimental paradigms), but three general procedures can be specified: (a) structure-function analysis, (b) sequence analysis, and (c) transition analysis. Sequence analysis includes structure-function analysis, and transition analysis includes sequence analysis. These procedures are approximated to varying degrees by extant methodologies and lines of research. We will provide examples to clarify each of these procedures, but no single example incorporates all of them.

Structure-Function Analysis

Any investigation begins with observations of the activities or behaviors of a system. Sets of these activities are related in that they are said to serve a certain function or goal. The first step in structure-function analysis is specification of the function to be studied. Next, a model (theory) is constructed to represent the inferred organization of activities involved in that function [*Overton,* 1975; *Reese and Overton,* 1970].

Structure-function analysis is commonly used by psychologists interested in the organization of behavioral systems. For example, *Bowlby* [1969] explicitly postulated that the function of certain infant and mother behaviors (e.g. signalling and approach behaviors) is the protection of the young from predators. Theories of attachment have been constructed to specify the organization of the behaviors that serve this function [*Bischof,* 1975; *Bowlby,* 1969]. *Klahr and Wallace* [1976, p. 29] employed the same strategy to model the organization of quantification processes which allow humans 'to determine how much or how many or how big'. Structure-function analysis is implicit in the work of information-processing psychologists like *Anderson* [1976], who has constructed models of the functions involved in linguistic and memorial activities (e.g. retrieval of information from memory to answer questions).

The *representation* of structure-function relationships can be critically important. Observations and measurements provide the raw material from which a representation (or theory or model) is constructed. Such representations are typically verbal, but mathematical, logical, or computer-simulational models can be used to attain greater explicitness, precision, or generality. The degree of understanding obtained is determined by the adequacy of the representations in generating and integrating further observations.

Since a behavioral system consists of several levels of activity, theories may be constructed to represent structure-function relationships at one or more levels. For example, the study of heuristics and planning may contribute as much to the understanding of problem-solving as a fine-grained analysis of visual pattern-matching, even though these two activities (functions) involve very different levels of cognitive analysis [*Newell and Simon,* 1972]. The key to a successful line of research often lies in the investigator's ability to specify the relations between the various levels of analysis. Postulation of levels of activity in no way implies a reductionistic framework. As *Weiss* [1969, pp. 10, 11] has noted:

'There is no phenomenon in a living system that is *not* molecular, but there is none that is *only* molecular, either. It is one thing not to see the forest for the trees, but then to go on and deny the reality of the forest is a more serious matter; for it is not just a case of myopia, but one of self-inflicted blindness.'

Sequence Analysis

Sequence Specification. Developmental analysis is concerned not with a single structure-function analysis but rather with a *series* of such analyses that specify the changing relationships between structure and function over time. Such a series of structure-function relationships is the basis for sequence analysis, the goal of which is to describe the nature of change by examining differences among successive states.

Due largely to the influence of *Piaget,* constructing a sequence of states to represent changing modes of system functioning is ubiquitous in the study of cognitive development. However, this strategy is not restricted to Piagetian researchers. Using an information-processing framework, for example, *Wilkinson* [1976] found evidence for two counting strategies that form an age-related sequence. The earlier strategy is appropriate for most cases but *not* for class inclusion tasks; the later strategy provides an adequate method for all instances in which counting is required. Similarly, *Siegler* [1976] and *Klahr and Siegler* [1979] outlined four sequential states in the acquisition of competence on balance-scale tasks, each state reflecting the questions, information, and decision rules employed by children operating at a particular level of performance. The procedure of sequence specification is exemplified in both cases: A series of structure-function analyses is performed, each structure (or strategy or stage) representing the mental activities and/or knowledge believed to be related to the function in question (e.g. counting, balance scale judgments) at different points in development.

Another approach has been undertaken by psychologists who employ computer simulation techniques [*Klahr,* 1973, 1976; *Klahr and Wallace,* 1976]. Their general method is (a) to analyze the performance of children at various levels of age and skill on a given task or set of tasks, (b) to represent performance at each of these levels in terms of hypothesized cognitive operations and processing parameters, (c) to incorporate these operations and parameters into operable computer programs, and (d) to test the validity of these representations by running the programs. If a program does not run successfully (i.e. if it fails completely or if it does not simulate observed performance to an acceptable degree), it is concluded that the hypothesized nature, sequence, and organization of the operations is inaccurate or insufficiently specified. If the program runs successfully, the investigators have some confidence that they have a 'sufficient' model of cognitive performance – one that at least deserves further specification, test, and modification. In a sense, the computer programs for each level of skill represent the sequence of cognitive development.

In the area of social cognition, *Selman's* [1975] work on role-taking provides an example of how a sequence analysis of developmental change might proceed. He conceptualizes role-taking as a developing process that can be characterized in terms of successive levels of organization. The first step in analyzing such a process is to specify the activity or function that is to be studied. *Selman* [1975] argued that the same function, the understanding of the relationship between one's own perspective and that of others, is the concern at each level of organization.

The second step is to perform a series of structure-function analyses. The resulting sequence must specify how the structure at each level interrelates with hierarchically superordinate and subordinate structures. *Selman and Byrne* [1974] derived the hypothesized sequence both logically (by noting parallels in cognitive and social development) and empirically (on the basis of their own and others' research). In defining the sequence of levels (structures), *Selman* [1975] equated differentiation to 'distinguishing perspectives' in role-taking and integration to coordinating or 'relating perspectives'. Six levels of perspective-taking were identified, each new level being characterized by the emergence of a new organizing principle. Thus, *Selman* attempted to specify the sequence of structures that characterizes the development of role-taking. His sequence constitutes a theoretical model that must be subjected to further empirical test: Are the inferred structures consistent with obtained data at each level? Is the sequence truly invariant?

In summary, a successful sequence analysis of developmental change involves showing that (a) the structure-function analysis at each successive stage adequately characterizes behavior, (b) the sequence of structures and behaviors is invariant, and (c) the successive stages conform to the definition of development presented earlier.

Parallels and the Concept of Main Sequence. Implicit in the developmental perspective is the assumption that development within similarly organized systems will have common properties [*Kaplan,* 1966; *Spencer,* 1862; *Werner,* 1957]. Thus, a thorough understanding of one system (and development within that system) may be useful in gaining an understanding of a second, less familiar system that is similar to the first in structure or function. This assumption gives rise to the strategy of 'looking for parallels'. The strategy is exemplified in a provoking and elegant paper by *Teitelbaum* [1977, pp. 10, 11], who argued that the experimental approach to understanding brain-behavior relationships has been quite successful in isolating the elements of behavioral phenomena (e.g. the reflex) but has been notably unsuccessful in recombining these elements into complex human or animal behavior. He proposed that:

> 'There is another method of synthesis, rather little exploited... It allows immediate useful application to complex behavior of any knowledge we have obtained about simpler, experimentally isolated behavior systems. It is 'synthesis by parallel', which in essence says that something new is like something else that is already familiar. A parallel is a similarity, and the more detailed it is the more confidence we have that the similarity is not mere coincidence. One uses this method from the conviction that nature is parsimonious: if a given phenomenon works in a particular fashion, it is likely that the same method is used to produce other phenomena which up to now we have not recognized as being the same. Therefore, look for a parallel.' (Reprinted by permission of Prentice-Hall, Inc., Englewood Cliffs, N.J.).

Parallels have been variously referred to as 'formal identities' [*Miller,* 1956], 'partial isomorphisms' [*Piaget,* 1971], 'formal parallelisms' [*Kaplan,* 1966], and 'analogies' [*Lorenz,* 1974; *Sechenov,* 1935]. Thus, looking for parallels is not a novel concept in psychology, and it is used in developmental analysis to facilitate sequence specification.

Consider the parallel between two phenomena in different domains: the recovery of manual grasping in adults following cerebral insult and the ontogeny of grasping in human newborns. In the literature of clinical neurology, *Seyffarth and Denny-Brown* [1948] identified two distinct types of grasping responses in patients with a variety of neurological disorders. One was the 'grasp reflex', in which the hand and fingers flex and hold in response to a specific contact stimulus. The other was the 'instinctive grasp reaction', a less stereotyped movement in which the hand orients and adjusts in order to grasp a contact stimulus object. *Seyffarth and Denny-Brown* [1948] postulated that the two types of responses are mediated by different, but related, cerebral mechanisms. Additional studies [*Denny-Brown* et al., 1949] further distinguished the 'traction response', which consists of flexion at all joints of a limb in response to a passive stretching of that limb. *Twitchell* [1951] identified these same three grasping automatisms in hemiplegic patients and, more importantly, discovered that they always appeared in an invariant sequence in the course of complete recovery: traction, grasp reflex, and instinctive grasp reaction.

In a different literature, that of motor skill acquisition, *Twitchell* [1965, 1970] demonstrated the existence of an invariant sequence in the development of voluntary control of grasping in infants – traction, grasp reflex, and instinctive grasp – the *same* sequence as that found in recovery from hemiplegia. *Twitchell* [1970] argued that the integration and sequencing of these three 'reflexes' are mediated at different levels of integration of the brain. The proprioceptive traction response is integrated at the level of the brain stem, the mechanism of the grasp reflex is integrated at a subcortical level, and the instinctive grasp reaction is integrated at the cortical level. The strategy of looking for parallels serves as a basis for integrating these two bodies of research, as well as accomplishing the broader objective of enhancing our understanding of neurological mechanisms involved in grasping.

Looking for parallels has also been a useful strategy in the study of perception. Knowledge about the ontogenesis of perception has been related to the study of 'microgenesis', or perceptual adaptation over a short period of time [*Flavell and Draguns,* 1957; *Werner,* 1957]. For example, *Held and Bossom* [1961] have stressed the importance of self-produced movement in both perceptual development in children and prism adaptation in adults. They have argued that 'an identical process underlies both the original development of coordination and its later adaptability to rearrangement' [*Held and Bossom,* 1961, p. 33]. More recently, *Rosinski* [1977, p. 120] suggested that learning a visual-motor coordination in development and relearning one in adaptation are not strictly identical, although 'the apparent homology between these processes generates a number of testable hypotheses about the course of development'.

Thus, the assumption about parallels in development permits an investigator to use current knowledge about the details of one sequence (e.g. ontogenesis) as a base from which to explore the details of a less familiar sequence (e.g. microgenesis). It is unlikely that any two sequences will ever be completely isomorphic, and an important aspect of using parallels is specification of the boundary conditions within which a hypothesized sequence is valid [*Miller,* 1956; *Oppenheimer,* 1956; *Slobodkin,* 1978]. However, the establishment and use of parallels as a heuristic (a) provides the investigator of an unfamiliar domain with suggestions for initial hypotheses, and (b) leads the investigator to diverse literatures where similar problems may have been explored (and perhaps resolved successfully).

Whereas a parallel is based on commonalities between two sequences, a *main sequence* consists of the abstracted characteristics of many parallel sequences. For example, *Siegel and White* [1975] tentatively have identified an invariant sequence in the development of spatial representations of large-scale environments among adults. Briefly, spatial representations begin as a set of associations between landmarks and later develop into a functional unit (the cognitive map). This sequence parallels invariant sequences observed in the development of spatial representation in children and is also consistent with sequences suggested by philosophical [*Bergson*, 1911] and neurological analyses [*Luria*, 1966; *Milner*, 1967].

Bruner [1970, 1973] has examined parallels in the development of motor control in adults and infants and described a very similar sequence of integration or 'modularization'. This sequence also parallels the type of change found by *Mandler* [1962, p. 417] in overlearning experiments with human adults and rats.

'The process unfolds in the following manner: First, the organism makes a series of discrete responses, often interrupted by incorrect ones. However, once errors are dropped out and the sequence of behavior becomes relatively stable – as in running a maze, speaking a word, reproducing a visual pattern – the various components of the total behavior required in the situation are "integrated". Integration refers to the fact that previously discrete parts of a sequence come to behave functionally as a unit; the whole sequence is elicited as a unit and behaves as a single component response has in the past; any part of it elicits the whole sequence.'

The common feature of all these sequences is that lower level units of organization – discrete responses and associations – become increasingly integrated into an overall, higher level organization, which in turn may become integrated into a still higher level. On the basis of the parallels among the sequences of change found in diverse areas of investigation, it is reasonable to postulate the operation of a main sequence. *Mandler's* [1962] phrase, 'from association to structure', is an appropriate label for this sequence.

The concept of main sequence is a direct outgrowth of the strategy of looking for parallels. The large number of similarities in sequences found in diverse bodies of research suggests the tantalizing possibility that development can occur only through certain sequences of organization. There may be certain design features of adapting systems in general, and the nervous system in particular, that would limit the range of possible sequences in development. Due to the fragmentary nature of our research on sequences, the question of whether there are one, many, or any main sequences remains moot [*Siegel and White*, 1975]. The critical point is that the notion of main sequence – of parallels in sequences of change across a variety of systems and time spans – is a potentially important conceptual tool for understanding change.

Transition Analysis

In developmental analysis, change is studied by first constructing successive states of organization (structure-function analysis). Inferences about the nature of change are then made by comparing the organization and order of these states (sequence analysis). Beyond description of sequence and generalization about the direction of change, the goal of transition analysis is to specify the principles, properties, or mechanisms of a system that result in self-regulation or self-modification. The distinction between representing states or stages and understanding transition has been made by *Simon* [1962, pp. 154, 155], who has advocated the use of computer programs to represent stages of organization in cognitive development.

'Having described a particular stage by a program, we would then face the task of discovering what additional information-processing mechanisms are needed to simulate developmental change – the transition from one stage to the next. That is, we would need to discover how the system could modify its own structure. Thus, the theory would have two parts – a program to describe performance at a particular stage and a learning program governing the transitions from stage to stage.'

Note that the emphasis is on *self*-regulation. In developmental psychology, answers to the question of how transition occurs range from statements about 'maturation' and 'cumulative learning' [*Gagné*, 1968] to those that invoke 'adaptive value'. From a developmental perspective, factors like maturation, antecedent events, and functional consequences (e.g. reinforcement) may be considered as *inputs* to the system, but the extent to which these inputs influence transition depends on the *organization* of the system and on the properties or mechanisms that regulate change in that system. Self-regulating properties or mechanisms coordinate factors such as maturation and experience [*Piaget*, 1971, 1977; *Piaget and Inhelder*, 1969].

Of the three procedures that make up developmental analysis, transition analysis is the most inclusive but it is also the one that has been specified least sufficiently. This lack of theoretical detail can be seen in the work of *Piaget*, whose writings constitute the most comprehensive theory of cognitive development to date. The regulatory concepts of assimilation, accommodation, and equilibration were introduced in *Piaget's* early writings in order to explain developmental transition. Unfortunately, with the possible exception of his analysis of sensorimotor development [*Piaget*, 1952], Piaget has not developed or formalized these concepts beyond a general, abstract level. For example, it is possible to describe *in general* what equilibration is and how it is essential to this theoretical scheme [*Piaget*, 1977]. However, the specific characteristics of the interplay between a given structure and environmental and maturational factors *in real time* is usually absent from the Piagetian analysis. The more specific interpretations of transition processes that derive from such an analysis [*Case*, 1978b] are at best debatable [see *Kuhn*, this volume].

An ideal transition analysis should fulfill several criteria. First, it should be based on a sequence analysis sufficiently detailed and accurate so that adequate mechanisms of transition can be inferred [*Klahr*, 1976]. Second, the mechanisms that regulate change must be specified in enough detail to (a) account for existing data in an unambiguous manner, and (b) lead to verifiable predictions about behavioral change.

The third criterion is that a theory about transitions should account for a *continued* and *constrained* course of development [*Kail and Bisanz*, 1982]. That is, the theory must explain more than a single change. Thus, explanations of invariant sequences require hypotheses about regulatory mechanisms that are *homeorhetic* [*Waddington*, 1969] rather than *homeostatic*. Whereas homeostasis involves maintenance of a fixed goal or equilibrium, homeorhesis involves the maintenance of a stable, consistent, and directional change in the system. Recognition that the 'goal' of developmental change is a path or sequence of states, not a single fixed state, implies that simple mechanisms of a homeostatic nature are insufficient for describing developmental regulations. Developmental theories ultimately will require an understanding of homeorhetic change. Moreover, the proposed regulatory mechanisms must be structured so that some paths are much more probable than others [*Lerner*, 1978].

Fourth, a theory of transition must define critical aspects or features of the environment that are important at different points in development. If development is considered to be the product of an interaction between internal structure and external events, then the nature of those external events must be specified. References to 'general experience' have limited utility [*Wohlwill*, 1973]. One implication of this criterion is that forms of 'task analysis' [*Resnick*, 1976; *Siegler*, 1976] will become increasingly important in isolating particular features of the environment that are important. Finally, a transition analysis should include an indication of the 'boundary conditions' (i.e. the range of environmental conditions and behavioral sequences) for which the proposed mechanism is operational.

No existing developmental theory includes a transition analysis that meets all of these criteria. However, some relatively recent approaches to the study of cognitive development attempt to provide a more adequate framework for the analysis of transition.

Whereas *Piaget* focused on the representation of knowledge at each of several stages of development, *Pascual-Leone* [1970] has undertaken to represent the regularities of change from stage to stage in terms of a single transition rule, the central feature of which is a quantitative, limited-capacity parameter, M, that increases linearly with age. Within the framework of the 'M-power' model, *Pascual-Leone* [1970] and *Case* [1974, 1978b] have attempted to integrate data on children's performance on such diverse tasks as memory span, class inclusion, and a series of successive motor acts. *Case* [1974] used this transition rule to construct process models of problem-solving at various age levels. Thus, *Pascual-Leone* and *Case* incorporate the sequence analyses of *Piaget* and have begun to formally analyze transition by (a) representing the regularities of transition with a single quantitative rule, and (b) integrating this rule into previously constructed models of cognitive functioning. The joint specification of sequence and a transition rule represents an effort to provide a more complete account of cognitive development [see *Halford and Wilson*, 1980, for a related approach].

A second approach to the study of transition is represented in *Bruner's* [1970, 1973] analysis of motor skill development in infancy.

As noted previously, motor skill development may be viewed as an instance of the 'association to structure' main sequence: Individual acts become differentiated from each other and integrated as units in higher-level organizations. *Bruner* has employed the concepts of *modularization* and *attentional capacity* to characterize the self-regulating properties of a system in transition. According to *Bruner*, a system requires attentional capacity for its operation, but the total amount of available capacity is always limited [*Kahneman*, 1973]. The emergence of new levels of behavioral integration is possible only when sufficient amounts of attentional capacity become available. Modularization is the process by which an individual act

'becomes less variable in latency and in execution time and more economical in expenditure of energy ... Modularization frees available information capacity for further use in task analysis, just by virtue of constituent subroutines requiring less attention ... But most important, given modularization and the reduction in attention necessary to regulate an act, that act can then be incorporated into a higher-order, longer-sequence act without requiring so much attention as to disrupt regulation of the higher-order act' [*Bruner*, 1973, p. 4].

The progression toward greater behavioral complexity requires simultaneous processes in which individual, lower-level acts become increasingly automated. This formulation is entirely consistent with *Jackson's* [1884] conceptualization of the organization and function of the human nervous system and with *Case's* [1978a] neo-Piagetian theory of cognitive development. The information-processing concepts of automaticity, modularization, and attentional capacity are potentially valuable constructs for understanding transitions in developing systems [*Kail and Bisanz*, 1982].

Evaluation of each of these approaches with respect to the criteria described previously is beyond the scope of this paper. None meets all the criteria. However, each represents a framework designed to provide an analysis of transition. Other approaches, such as the use of catastrophe theory [*Klahr and Wallace*, 1976; *Saari*, 1977], may prove to be useful. As the focus on problems of transition become more clearly defined in psychology, artificial intelligence, and other areas, more adequate concepts and procedures for transition analysis will be brought to bear on the problem.

Conclusion

In this paper we have tried to specify a contemporary form of developmental analysis, a distinct perspective and set of procedures that provide heuristics for the study of psychological change. Psychologists are becoming more and more concerned with change in organized systems. For example, much contemporary theory and research in cognitive psychology has been focused on the performance of well-practiced and 'competent' cognitive systems (typically in adults). However, there is a growing interest in the *acquisition* of complex knowledge and skill [*Anderson,* 1981; *Hayes-Roth,* 1977], especially in the study of language [*Anderson,* 1976] and problem-solving [*Greeno,* 1977; *Neches and Hayes,* 1978]. At the same time, there is a growing awareness of a lack of models in human experimental psychology for conceptualizing change [*Rabbitt,* 1981].

The growing interest in psychological change is by no means limited to the study of human cognition. While research on the topic of behavioral regulatory mechanisms in normal adult animals continues to be important, psychobiologists have begun to study *changes* in these mechanisms in ontogeny and during the course of recovery following brain damage [*Marshall and Teitelbaum,* 1974]. As psychological theory and research proceed toward the goal of understanding complex behavioral change, more adequate and sophisticated procedures of inquiry will be needed.

With increasing emphasis on behavioral change, we might expect developmental psychology to be at the forefront of these inquiries with an arsenal of conceptual and empirical tools for analyzing change. What we find instead is a proliferation of structure-function analyses and sequence analyses, along with some very general discussions about the nature of development [*Kitchener,* 1978, 1980; *Lerner,* 1978, 1980]. Noticeably lacking are detailed and comprehensive analyses of transition that meet the various criteria we have described.

Why does developmental psychology lack adequate analyses of transition? A thorough discussion is beyond the scope of this chapter, but we briefly suggest four possible reasons. First, researchers often describe states or sequences in a way that is not sufficiently precise and detailed to permit inferences about specific characteristics of transition from and to these states [*Kail and Bisanz,* 1982; *Klahr,* 1976]. At best, vague state or sequence descriptions can lead only to very general conclusions about transition. Second, developmental psychologists often fail to use the method of 'looking for parallels' to find possible main sequences. Identification of such sequences across different phenomena highlights the components of structure and function that are particularly relevant to analyses of transition [*Siegel and White*, 1975; *Werner*, 1957] and thus should facilitate these analyses.

Third, developmental psychologists have been highly reluctant to advance specific, if speculative, ideas about transition. Consequently, analyses of sequences are generated without reference to theories of transition. As *Klahr and Siegler* [1979] noted, sequence analyses should be *developmentally tractable*, that is, successive states in the sequence should be represented so that the links between states are feasible. Judgments of feasibility, however, require explicit theories of transition. We suspect that highly detailed theories of transition, even if wrong, are more useful at the present stage of theoretical development than more general theories. Fourth and finally, advances in the analysis of transitions require conceptual frameworks that allow sequences to be represented with great flexibility and precision. Developmental psychologists must be willing to abandon frameworks that do not meet these criteria and adopt others that appear more promising. Approaches associated traditionally with other disciplines (such as biology) or other areas of psychology (such as information processing) may be appropriate.

These four problems are not likely to be addressed in a coherent and comprehensive way as long as developmental psychologists do not share a common agenda, at least at a general level. Developmental analysis provides a framework of goals and general methods that are appropriate to a wide variety of pursuits within developmental psychology and would serve to focus research and theory on the important problem of understanding transition.

Although the important tasks of identifying classes of behavioral change and clarifying the mechanisms of transition are incomplete [*Flavell*, 1971, 1972; *Neches and Hayes*, 1978], it is clear that development, defined in terms of 'differentiation and integration', constitutes only one class of change, at best. We defined development in this limited way because such a definition has a degree of historical precedence and was useful in explicating general procedures for the study of change. Although the terms 'differentiation' and 'integration' have been useful in the past, they are too imprecise and limited. A brief survey of current work confirms that more useful and varied concepts are being derived to characterize common sequences of psychological change. For example, developmental psychologists who adopt an information-processing perspective have shown how the concepts of attentional capacity and automatization can be useful to explain certain sequences of change [*Case*, 1978a; *Kail and Bisanz*, 1982; *Pascual-Leone*, 1970]. *Klahr and Wallace* [1976] suggested that processes for detecting regularities and eliminating redundancies are necessary properties for self-modifying systems in cognitive development. *Kail and Bisanz* [1982] reviewed several sequences of cognitive change and proposed a 'transitional system' to account for certain characteristics of change. This system includes processes that detect both inconsistencies and recurrent regularities, processes that modify knowledge structures, and a dynamic interchange between limited attentional resources and the contents of knowledge that propels developmental change in the direction of increasing *efficiency* and *sufficiency*. *Lawler* [1981] describes processes of *specialization, refinement, control elevation*, and *perspective correlation* in the context of a child's developing skills in arithmetic. These processes are similar to 'differentiation' and 'integration' in some ways, but the rich empirical descriptions and theoretical context make the definitions of these processes clearer and more explicit. Not all of the concepts described above can be subsumed under the terms 'differentiation' and 'integration', although certain relationships can be suggested.

At this point in the construction of developmental theories, adherence to a highly exclusive concept of development is unwarranted. Identification of invariant sequences and possible main sequences, along with analyses of transition that meet the criteria described in the preceding section, is the important goal. As sequence and transition analyses become more precise, the features that distinguish classes of change should become clearer.

Although the elements of developmental analysis are not in themselves new, when considered as a whole they provide a rich framework for the study of change. To the extent that the focus of theory and research is on *any* type of change in a system, the procedures of developmental analysis – structure-function, sequence, and transition analyses, as well as the strategy of looking for parallels – provide a useful framework for investigators. Such an approach is compatible, for example, with the goals of the emerging field of instructional psychology

[*Glaser*, 1981; *Lesgold* et al., 1978; *Resnick*, 1981]. It has been argued that instructional theory must be directed toward characterizing both (a) initial and subsequent states of the learner's knowledge, and (b) the conditions or mechanisms that influence transition from state to state [*Glaser*, 1976]. Whereas developmental analysis is primarily a descriptive enterprise, instructional psychology is prescriptive in the sense that a major goal is to optimize the acquisition of knowledge and skills. In spite of this difference in agenda, the procedures developed by psychologists interested in analyzing sequences of change should prove useful to scientists concerned with optimizing change.

Viewing problems of interest from the perspective of developmental analysis can provide a vehicle for meaningful dialogue between researchers within developmental psychology, as well as between developmental psychologists and researchers in such traditionally diverse areas as cognitive psychology, clinical neurology, psychobiology, and other domains in the behavioral and social sciences. Much is to be gained by looking at changes in psychological phenomena as legitimate problems for a more broadly conceived psychology of development.

Summary

In this paper we specify a contemporary form of 'developmental analysis', a distinct perspective and set of procedures for the study of behavioral change. Developmental analysis has its roots in the 'development hypothesis' of *Herbert Spencer*, is integral to the work of *Jean Piaget* and *Heinz Werner*, and has an extended history of employment in a variety of scientific contexts. Examples from contemporary and historical research and theory are provided to illustrate the characteristics of this perspective and the general procedures generated from it, including structure-function, sequence, and transition analyses, as well as the strategy of looking for parallels. Benefits of developmental analysis as an agenda for research in developmental psychology are argued to be considerable. The framework could serve to define the field as a subdiscipline with shared goals and methods; in so doing it could make a developmental approach increasingly central to investigations in diverse areas of psychology.

Acknowledgement

Preparation of this paper was made possible in part by NSF/NIE Grant No. SEB-7912743 to the first author and a grant from the Natural Sciences and Engineering Research Council of Canada to the second author. The third author was supported by the

Centre for the Study of Mental Retardation, University of Alberta. The authors are grateful to *N. Harway, R. Kail, G. Vesonder, J. Voss,* and *S.H. White* for comments on earlier versions of this paper.

References

Anderson, J.R.: Language, memory, and thought (Erlbaum, Hillsdale 1976).
Anderson, J.R.: Cognitive skills and their acquisition (Erlbaum, Hillsdale 1981).
Bergson, H.: Creative evolution (Holt, New York 1911).
Bergson, H.: The creative mind (Philosophical Library, New York 1946); originally published 1922.
Bertalanffy, L. von: Robots, men and minds (Braziller, New York 1967).
Bertalanffy, L. von: General system theory (Braziller, New York 1968).
Bischof, N.: A systems approach toward the functional connections of attachment and fear. Child Dev. *46:* 801–817 (1975).
Blumenthal, A.L.: The process of cognition (Prentice-Hall, Englewood Cliffs 1977).
Bowlby, J.: Attachment and loss, vol. 1 (Hogarth Press, London 1969).
Bruner, J.S.: The growth of structure and skill; in Connolly, Mechanisms of motor skill development (Academic Press, London 1970).
Bruner, J.S.: Organization of early skilled action. Child Dev. *44:* 1–11 (1973).
Case, R.: Structures and strictures: some functional limitations on the course of cognitive growth. Cognitive Psychol. *6:* 544–573 (1974).
Case, R.: Intellectual development from birth to adolescence: a neo-Piagetian interpretation; in Siegler, Children's thinking: What develops? (Erlbaum, Hillsdale 1978a).
Case, R.: Piaget and beyond: toward a developmentally based theory and technology of instruction; in Glaser, Advances in instructional psychology, vol. 1 (Erlbaum, Hillsdale 1978b).
Denny-Brown, D.; Twitchell, T.E.; Saenz-Arroyo, L.: The nature of spasticity resulting from cerebral lesions. Trans. Am. neurol. Ass. *74:* 108–113 (1949).
Fischer, K.W.: A theory of cognitive development: the control and construction of hierarchies of skills. Psychol. Rev. *87:* 477–531 (1980).
Fishbein, H.D.: Evolution, development, and children's learning (Goodyear, Pacific Palisades 1976).
Flavell, J.H.: Stage-related properties of cognitive development. Cognitive Psychol. *2:* 421–453 (1971).
Flavell, J.H.: An analysis of cognitive-developmental sequences. Genetic Psychol. Monogr. *86:* 279–350 (1972).
Flavell, J.H.; Draguns, J.: A microgenetic approach to perception and thought. Psychol. Bull. *54:* 197–217 (1957).
Gagné, R.M.: Contributions of learning to human development. Psychol. Rev. *75:* 177–191 (1968).
Gentner, D.: Evidence for the psychological reality of semantic components: the verbs of possession; in Norman, Rumelhart, and the LNR Research Group, Explorations in cognition (Freeman, San Francisco 1975).

Glaser, R.: Components of a psychology of instruction: toward a science of design. Rev. educ. Res. *46:* 1-24 (1976).

Glaser, R.: Instructional psychology: past, present, and future. Pädagog. Stud. *58:* 111-122 (1981).

Greeno, J.G.: Process of understanding in problem solving; in Castellan, Pisoni, Potts, Cognitive theory, vol. 2 (Erlbaum, Hillsdale 1977).

Grinder, R.: The history of genetic psychology (Wiley, New York 1968).

Halford, G.S.; Wilson, W.H.: A category theory approach to cognitive development. Cognitive Psychol. *12:* 356-411 (1980).

Hayes-Roth, B.: Evolution of cognitive structures and processes. Psychol. Rev. *84:* 260-278 (1977).

Held, R.; Bossom, J.: Neonatal deprivation and adult rearrangement: complementary techniques for analyzing plastic sensory-motor coordination. J. comp. physiol. Psychol. *54:* 33-37 (1961).

Hull, C.L.: Principles of behavior (Appleton Century Crofts, New York 1943).

Jackson, J.H.: On the duality of the brain; in Taylor, The selected writings of John Hughlings Jackson, vol. 1 (Basic Books, New York 1958); originally published in Medical Press and Circular, 1874.

Jackson, J.H.: Evolution and dissolution of the nervous system; in Taylor, The selected writings of John Hughlings Jackson, vol. 2 (Basic Books, New York 1958); from the Croonian Lectures, originally published 1884.

Jerison, H.J.: Paleoneurology and the evolution of mind. Scient. Am. *234:* 90-101 (1976).

Kahneman, D.: Attention and effort (Prentice-Hall, Englewood Cliffs 1973).

Kail, R.; Bisanz, J.: Information processing and cognitive development; in Reese, Advances in child development and behavior, vol. 17 (Academic Press, New York 1982).

Kaplan, B.: The study of language in psychiatry; in Arieti, American handbook of psychiatry, vol. 3 (Basic Books, New York 1966).

Kaplan, B.: Mediations on genesis. Hum. Dev. *10:* 65-87 (1967).

Kitchener, R.F.: Epigenesis: the role of biological models in developmental psychology. Hum. Dev. *21:* 141-160 (1978).

Kitchener, R.F.: Predetermined versus probabilistic epigenesis: a reply to Lerner. Hum. Dev. *23:* 73-76 (1980).

Klahr, D.: An information processing approach to the study of cognitive development; in Pick, Minnesota symposia on child psychology, vol. 7 (University of Minnesota Press, Minneapolis 1973).

Klahr, D.: Steps toward the simulation of intellectual development; in Resnick, The nature of intelligence (Erlbaum, Hillsdale 1976).

Klahr, D.; Siegler, R.S.: The representation of children's knowledge; in Reese, Lipsitt, Advances in child development and behavior, vol. 14 (Academic Press, New York 1979).

Klahr, D.; Wallace, J.G.: Cognitive development: an information-processing view (Erlbaum, Hillsdale 1976).

Kohlberg, L.: The development of children's orientations toward a moral order. 1. Sequence in the development of moral thought. Vita hum. *6:* 11-33 (1963).

Kurtines, W.; Grief, E.B.: The development of moral thought: review and evaluations of Kohlberg's approach. Psychol. Bull. *81:* 453-470 (1974).

Lawler, R.W.: The progressive construction of mind. Cognitive Sci. 5: 1–30 (1981).
Lerner, R.M.: Nature, nurture, and dynamic interaction. Hum. Dev. 21: 1–10 (1978).
Lerner, R.M.: Concepts of epigenesis: descriptive and explanatory issues, a critique of Kitchener's comments. Hum. Dev. 23: 63–72 (1980).
Lesgold, A.M.; Pellegrino, J.W.; Fokkema, S.; Glaser, R.: Cognitive psychology and instruction (Plenum Press, New York 1978).
Lorenz, K.Z.: Analogy as a source of knowledge in science. Science 185: 229–234 (1974).
Luria, A.R.: Higher cortical functions in man (Basic Books, New York 1966).
MacLean, P.D.: The triune brain, emotion, and scientific bias; in Schmitt, The neurosciences: second study program (Rockefeller University Press, New York 1970).
Mandler, G.: From association to structure. Psychol. Rev. 69: 415–427 (1962).
Marshall, J.F.; Teitelbaum, P.: Further analysis of sensory inattention following lateral hypothalamic damage in rats. J. comp. physiol. Psychol. 86: 375–395 (1974).
McCandless, B.R.; Geis, M.F.: Current trends in developmental psychology; in Reese, Advances in child development and behavior, vol. 10 (Academic Press, New York 1975).
Miller, J.G.: Toward a general theory for the behavioral sciences; in White, The state of the social sciences (University of Chicago Press, Chicago 1956).
Milner, E.: Human neural and behavioral development (Thomas, Springfield 1967).
Murphy, G.; Kovach, J.K.: Historical introduction to modern psychology; 3rd ed. (Harcourt Brace Jovanovich, New York 1972).
Neches, R.; Hayes, J.R.: Progress towards a taxonomy of strategy transformations; in Lesgold, Pellegrino, Fokkema, Glaser, Cognitive psychology and instruction (Plenum Press, New York 1978).
Newell, A.; Simon, H.A.: Human problem solving (Prentice-Hall, Englewood Cliffs 1972).
Novikoff, A.B.: The concept of integrative levels and biology. Science 101: 209–215 (1945).
Oppenheimer, R.: Analogy in science. Am. Psychol. 11: 127–135 (1956).
Overton, W.F.: General systems, structure and development; in Riegel, Rosenwald, Structure and transformation: developmental and historical aspects (Wiley, New York 1975).
Pascual-Leone, J.: A mathematical model for the transition rule in Piaget's developmental stages. Acta psychol. 63: 301–345 (1970).
Pattee, H.: Hierarchy theory (Braziller, New York 1973).
Piaget, J.: The origins of intelligence in children (International Universities Press, New York 1952).
Piaget, J.: Structuralism (Basic Books, New York 1970).
Piaget, J.: Biology and knowledge (University of Chicago Press, Chicago 1971).
Piaget, J.: Problems of equilibration; in Appel, Goldberg, Topics in cognitive development, vol. 1 (Plenum Press, New York 1977).
Piaget, J.; Inhelder, B.: The psychology of the child (Basic Books, New York 1969).
Rabbitt, P.M.A.: Cognitive psychology needs models for changes in performance with old age; in Long, Baddeley, Attention and performance, vol. IX (Erlbaum, Hillsdale 1981).
Reese, H.W.; Overton, W.F.: Models of development and theories of development; in Goulet, Baltes, Life-span developmental psychology: research and theory (Academic Press, New York 1970).

Resnick, L.B.: Task analysis in instructional design: some cases from mathematics; in Klahr, Cognition and instruction (Erlbaum, Hillsdale 1976).
Resnick, L.B.: Instructional psychology; in Rosenzweig, Porter, Annual review of psychology, vol. 32 (Annual Reviews, Palo Alto 1981).
Ribot, T.: The psychology of attention; 6th revised ed. (Open Court, Chicago 1911).
Riegel, K.F.: The dialectics of human development. Am. Psychol. *31:* 689–700 (1976).
Rosinski, R.R.: The development of visual perception (Goodyear, Santa Monica 1977).
Rozin, P.: The evolution of intelligence and access to the cognitive unconscious; in Sprague, Epstein, Progress in psychobiology and physiological psychology (Academic Press, New York 1976).
Saari, D.G.: A qualitative model for the dynamics of cognitive processes. J. math. Psychol. *15:* 145–168 (1977).
Sechenov, I.M.: Selected works (State Publishing House, Moscow 1935).
Selman, R.L.: The relation of social perspective-taking to moral development: analytic and empirical approaches. Proc. Meet. of the Eastern Psychological Association, New York 1975.
Selman, R.L.; Byrne, D.F.: A structural-developmental analysis of levels of role taking in middle childhood. Child Dev. *45:* 803–806 (1974).
Seyffarth, H.; Denny-Brown, D.: The grasp reflex and the instinctive grasp reaction. Brain *71:* 109–183 (1948).
Siegel, A.W.: 'Remembering' is alive and well (and even thriving) in empiricism; in Datan, Reese, Life-span developmental psychology: dialectical perspectives on experimental research (Academic Press, New York 1977).
Siegel, A.W.; Kirasic, K.C.; Kail, R.V.: Stalking the elusive cognitive map: the development of children's representations of geographic space; in Wohlwill, Altman, Human behavior and environment, vol. 3 (Plenum Press, New York 1978).
Siegel, A.W.; White, S.H.: The development of spatial representations of large-scale environments; in Reese, Advances in child development and behavior, vol. 10 (Academic Press, New York 1975).
Siegler, R.S.: Three aspects of cognitive development. Cognitive Psychol. *8:* 481–520 (1976).
Simon, H.A.: An information processing theory of intellectual development. Monogr. Soc. Res. Child Dev. *27:* serial No. 82 (1962).
Simon, H.A.: The organization of complex systems; in Pattee, Hierarchy theory (Braziller, New York 1973).
Slobodkin, L.B.: Nothing but? Sciences *18:* 22–24 (1978).
Smith, E.E.: Theories of semantic memory; in Estes, Handbook of learning and cognitive processes, vol. 6 (Erlbaum, Hillsdale 1978).
Spencer, H.: First principles; 6th ed. (Appleton, New York 1900); originally published 1862.
Spencer, H.: Principles of biology, vol. 1 (Williams & Norgate, London 1899); originally published 1864.
Spencer, H.: The principles of psychology, vol. 2 (Appleton, New York 1896); originally published 1870.
Spencer, H.: An autobiography, vol. 2 (Williams & Norgate, London 1904).
Spiker, C.C.: The concept of development: relevant and irrelevant issues. Monogr. Soc. Res. Child Dev. *31:* serial No. 107 (1966).

Sutherland, J.W.: A general systems philosophy for the social and behavioral sciences (Braziller, New York 1973).

Teitelbaum, P.: Levels of integration of the operant; in Honig, Staddon, Handbook of operant behavior (Prentice-Hall, Englewood Cliffs 1977).

Twitchell, T.E.: The restoration of motor function following hemiplegia in man. Brain 74: 443–480 (1951).

Twitchell, T.E.: The automatic grasping responses in infants. Neuropsychologia 3: 247–259 (1965).

Twitchell, T.E.: Reflex mechanisms and the development of prehension; in Connolly, Mechanisms of motor skill development (Academic Press, New York 1970).

Waddington, C.H.: The theory of evolution today; in Koestler, Smythies, Beyond reductionism (Beacon Press, Boston 1969).

Weiss, P.A.: The living system: determinism stratified; in Koestler, Smythies, Beyond reductionism (Beacon Press, Boston 1969).

Werner, H.: Comparative psychology of mental development (International Universities Press, New York 1948).

Werner, H.: The concept of development from a comparative and organismic point of view; in Harris, The concept of development (University of Minnesota Press, Minneapolis 1957).

Werner, H.; Kaplan, B.: The developmental approach to cognition: Its relevance to the psychological interpretation of anthropological and ethnolinguistic data. Am. Anthrop. 58: 866–880 (1956).

White, S.H.: The learning theory approach; in Mussen, Carmichael's manual of child psychology (Wiley, New York 1970).

White, S.H.; Siegel, A.W.: Cognitive development: the new inquiry. Young Child. 31: 425–435 (1976).

Wilkinson, A.: Counting strategies and semantic analysis as applied to class inclusion. Cognitive Psychol. 8: 64–85 (1976).

Wohlwill, J.F.: Methodology and research strategy in the study of developmental change; in Goulet, Baltes, Life-span developmental psychology: research and theory (Academic Press, New York 1970).

Wohlwill, J.F.: The concept of experience: S or R? Hum. Dev. 16: 90–107 (1973).

On the Dual Executive and Its Significance in the Development of Developmental Psychology

Deanna Kuhn

Harvard University, Cambridge, Mass., USA

In North America in the early 1980s, we find the field of developmental psychology in a transitional period in its own development. Compelled to characterize the major dimensions of this transition in a sentence or two, one would probably cite on the theoretical front the growing disillusionment with *Piaget* and the increasing utilization of information-processing models in work on cognitive development. On the methodological front, one might cite a decreasing confidence in laboratory studies and an increasing concern for how the academic discipline should relate to real-world decisions of policy and practice.

If this is the case, it is perhaps a fruitful time for the field to engage in some conscious reflection on itself – retrospective and prospective – and it is toward this objective that this essay is directed. To anticipate somewhat its conclusion, the present essay makes an argument against faddism in psychology. This term may be more pejorative in its connotation than my meaning warrants, for the faddism to which I refer is not a thoroughly bad thing, serving in many ways perhaps to keep the field going. It is probably accurate to say, in any case, that the field of psychology as a whole, and developmental psychology in particular, have tended to indulge in faddism. Paralleling that tendency has been a tendency on the part of psychology not to view itself within the context of its own history.

It is not difficult to point to examples of faddism in American developmental psychology. The conservation training studies of the 1960s and early 1970s are one remarkable example. A more recent example is the current enthusiasm toward identifying the competencies of the preschool child. This latter work is not without its theoretical motivation and significance, but like the conservation training studies and the laboratory studies of imitation of the 1960s and numerous other examples, it is as a research strategy that it has gained its popularity. In contrast, the faddism I am concerned with in the present paper is I would argue of a more serious sort, having to do with a field's theories, more than its methods.

A number of assumptions, biases if you like, will underlie my approach to the topic, and I shall attempt to make those explicit at the outset. First, the discussion that follows will render apparent my commitment to theory itself – a belief in its value and indeed necessity if the field is to progress. I happen to think *Kurt Lewin* was right in claiming that there is nothing so practical as a good theory, but even within the narrower domain of academic inquiry, I regard theorizing, of both the cosmic and local variety, as an essential part of inquiry, functioning both to direct empirical investigation and to ascribe meanings to its outcomes.

Following from this commitment to theory is a commitment to what I will refer to as the enterprise of metatheory, or metatheorizing. By this I mean the continuing and self-conscious examination of one's own theorizing and modes of inquiry that accompany it. The value of this metatheorizing does not, in my view, stem from the relative youth of the social sciences, such that they have not yet gotten it straight exactly what they are doing, i.e. are in a 'prescientific' stage of formulating the rules that will characterize their discipline's activities. Rather, it arises from a recognition that both theory and method evolve (in interrelated fashion), and to fully understand what one is thinking or doing at the moment, and in what directions this thought or activity might be evolving, requires contemplation of both, from a dynamic, historical perspective.

The history of theory in American developmental psychology is, strictly speaking, rather short. The origins of modern developmental psychology can be traced to the child study movement that flourished at the beginning of this century, a movement characterized by *White* [1979] as a 'sprawling, polyglot empiricism'. Some cosmic theorizing also existed during this period, but it remained, at very best, loosely related to the field's research activities. The original child study movement matured into the child psychology of the 1930s, but it retained its characteristics of being separated from the academic discipline of psychology and focused on practical issues of child management and welfare. The maturationist doctrine, that originated with *G. Stanley Hall* but became most well-known in the work of *Gesell,* enjoyed a brief period in the limelight, but even *Gesell's* work was presented and received with more of an eye towards its practical utilization than its theoretical significance. It is fair to say, then, that when the learning theory that had come to dominate the mainstream of academic psychology embraced child psychology, this was the first time the activities of the field became seriously linked to any overarching theoretical framework.

Whether child psychology was saved or devoured by this embracement depends on one's point of view. It can be argued that learning theorists did (and continue to) employ child subjects out of convenience, to investigate issues of relevance only to the theory itself (as opposed to children or development). Others would hold that learning theory offered the first productive means of conceptualizing the phenomena of child development. In either event, the dual influences of Hullian learning theory and Skinnerian behavior theory in large part shaped the enterprise known as child or developmental psychology through the 1940s and 1950s.

The last two decades have seen extraordinarily rapid evolution in the theoretical paradigms guiding inquiry in American developmental psychology, relative to the comparatively brief and uncomplicated theoretical history that preceded this period. In the present essay, I examine the evolution of theory in one segment of the field of developmental psychology, that of cognitive development, over the last couple of decades, using the theoretical formulations of *Case* [1978a, b] as a focal point for this analysis.

From Piaget to Information-Processing

Advocates and detractors alike will agree that the single most prominent figure in the field of cognitive development during the past two decades has been *Piaget*. It is perhaps true that the field was in many ways ripe for its 'discovery' of *Piaget,* as historical reviews of the field have noted. It was time for 'Rediscovering the Mind of the Child', as *Martin* titled his 1959/60 article. Nevertheless, the rapid growth in the awareness and popularity of *Piaget's* work in this country was indeed remarkable. In the space of a very few years, *Piaget's* work travelled a route from relative obscurity to attain what in many circles became a sweeping and largely uncritical embracement and in others a more reserved but solid respect.

In 1969, the American Psychological Association awarded *Piaget* its Distinguished Scientific Contribution Award, attesting to the recognition his work had attained and his popularity at that point in time. Given this event, and the history of the decade leading up to it, it is all the more remarkable, then, that just a decade later, at the end of the 1970s, *Piaget's* theory seems all wrong to many developmental psychologists, such that a leading, and notably level-headed, spokesman in the field has been led to remark about what has been regarded as the foundation of *Piaget's* theory, the concept of stage: 'My own hunch is that the concept of stage will not, in fact, figure importantly in future scientific work on cognitive growth' [*Flavell*, 1977, p. 249].

Interestingly, one can even trace this historical rise and fall as it has filtered through to applied fields distinct from but significantly influenced by mainstream academic psychology. In the field of children's advertising, for example, an article in the 1979 volume of the series *Current Issues and Research in Advertising* is titled 'Television Advertising and Young Children: Piaget Reconsidered'. Its author laments the domination of this field by *'Piaget* and his assumption of stage-dependent cognitive skills'. He says:

> 'Many important policy questions regarding television advertising to children are now premised on this assumption. Consumer research has been responsible for this. Adopting Piaget's theory from the very outset, it has maintained an uncritical acceptance of concepts which should have come under greater scrutiny' [*Chestnut*, 1979, pp. 12, 13].

Chestnut goes on to describe how developmental psychology itself has been much more critical of *Piaget* than has his own consumer research field, citing papers by *Brainerd, Gelman, Flavell,* and others. The current view in psychology, he concludes, is that 'the young child is developing, but can no longer be defined by stage'. This calls into question, *Chestnut* [1979] believes, the prevailing view that children's cognitive development imposes limitations on their comprehension of advertising, and he criticizes those in his own field for not having 'kept pace with an increasingly critical and sophisticated view of *Piaget's* theory and the implications of that view for the information processing abilities of young children'.

Is *Piaget's* theory primarily a theory of stages? I shall argue in a later section that it is not. For a probably complex set of reasons, however, American developmental psychology has focused on Piagetian theory as a doctrine of stages. There has been some considerable attention paid to the question of the mechanism of development of those stages, and in particular whether the doctrine of stages puts *Piaget* into a maturationist camp, with followers of *Piaget* tending toward the sanctimonious on occasion in their attempts to explain how *Piaget's* stages reflect another alternative than biological determinism to colleagues who they believe have understood *Piaget* less well. Nevertheless, it is the existence of those stages in the child's development, rather than the nature of their origin, that has been the center of attention.

Why this is so is not completely clear. One can point to a number of possible explanations, but there are also some reasons to think that the theory might have been received differently. One can rather easily accept the surge in popularity of *Piaget* in this country as a response to the excesses of the behaviorist doctrine that was at its height at the time. *Kessen* [quoted in *Senn,* 1975, p. 54] has remarked of this turn of events that *Piaget* '... clearly, in a sense, rescued us from many of the holes we were about to dig ourselves into', although *Kessen* went on to comment, 'He could have done it 30 years earlier, and why American psychologists suddenly became attached to him in the fifties instead of the thirties or forties is another historical mystery' [*Senn,* 1975, p. 54]. In any event, once it happened, one might have expected that it was the 'rediscovery of the child's mind' that *Piaget* would come to stand for.

There were evidently stronger forces, however, leading American psychology's assimilation of *Piaget* in a different direction. The doctrine of stages was in some sense the most *visible* aspect of *Piaget's* theory. It may also have been perceived as the most empirically testable, thus permitting the theory to be assimilated into the positivist view of science that prevailed at the time. Furthermore, the doctrine of stages no doubt attracted the attention of American developmental psychologists in that it represented a challenge, and what looked like an empirically testable one, to prevailing empiricist theories, implying as it did both the inevitability of the sequence of stages and their resistance to environmental influence.

What then has led in the space of a very few years to current disenchantment with *Piaget's* theory of stages? It would be impossible here to review, or even cite, the by now sizable number of studies making claims to have refuted some aspect of *Piaget's* theory. The literature critical of *Piaget* is diverse in both approach and scope, and has never been marshalled into a single, connected argument against the theory. In what follows, I shall attempt to portray in a brief space the major lines of the argument someone critical of *Piaget's* theory of stages might make.

The argument would be likely to be some combination of conceptual analysis suggesting that the theory is untestable or meaningless and empirical analysis suggesting that it is false. The major argument on the conceptual front is that stage theory is inherently untestable, and accordingly of little scientific merit, the reason being that there exists no means of empirically assessing the presence of a stage independent of the behaviors that are alleged to be a manifestation of that stage. Accordingly, assertions of the form 'S does x because she is at stage X' become empty circularities.

If one accepts this argument, it follows that if the construct of stage is to be of any value, stage must be regarded not as an independent predictor of behavior but rather as some form of 'explanation' or 'abstract description' of a set of behaviors. If this is granted, how, then, does one evaluate the correctness of *Piaget's* descriptions? Presumably one would look first to criteria established by *Piaget* himself as the necessary characteristics of stages, notably the criteria of discontinuity and 'structured wholeness'.

The discontinuity criterion has a range of interpretations. One has to do with the idea of qualitative versus quantitative change. This distinction has by now been recognized, however, to be dependent on the level of analysis. Colors, for example, differ from one another qualitatively at one level of analysis but quantitatively at another. To say for sure, then, whether two behaviors differ from one another qualitatively or quantitatively depends on the conceptual structure in terms of which the behaviors are regarded. This underlying 'structure', however, in the case of behaviors alleged to be stage manifestations, is exactly what one is trying to confirm! A more empirical, as opposed to conceptual, interpretation of discontinuity centers around the abruptness of stage-related change: If stages are discontinuous structures, the transition from one stage to the next must take place abruptly rather than gradually. One can argue the correctness of the interpretation, but in any case the empirical evidence, and there is a substantial amount in this case, is overwhelmingly on the side of gradualness, for every type of conceptual or behavior change that has been examined.

The 'structured whole' criterion has met with an even wider range of interpretations and modes of evaluation. The core of the argument is that behaviors alleged to be manifestations of a single structure ought to emerge synchronously. A substantial amount of empirical evidence has accumulated showing a lack of such synchrony. One can argue that the tests are unfair, for example that they have not equated for more superficial performance demands across tasks, but in any case the situation stands that there has been no impressive positive evidence in support of synchrony. Even more damaging to the 'structured whole' criterion is evidence not just that behaviors indicative of a given stage emerge at slightly different times but that some elements of a stage can be detected well before the age appropriate to their alleged stage level while others do not appear until the child is well advanced into the stage following the one in question. Perspective-taking, for example, to cite one of the most well-studied instances, is alleged in Piagetian theory to appear with the development of concrete operations. Empirical data, however, show that certain forms of perspective-taking are present in preoperational children while other forms are not mastered until some time during the stage of formal operations. In the face of such evidence, the concept of 'global stage' (e.g. concrete operations) appears to lose much of its force, in as much as some of its defining properties, or some forms of its defining properties, are evidently within the child's competence prior to the advent of the stage while others remain beyond the child's competence even after the stage has been attained.

Further arguments against the global stage, or structured whole, concept come from the experimental 'training' literature. If certain elements or behavioral manifestations that go towards defining a stage can be singled out and successfully trained by relatively superficial external teaching, this casts doubt on the claim that these individual elements are manifestations of a 'structured whole'. One can question the 'genuineness' of these experimentally induced attainments, but at the very least the child displays at least some of the superficial behaviors characteristic of the higher stage; to make such an argument, one thus needs to appeal to some less behaviorally anchored criteria of stage, and it is problematic how these should be defined and measured.

Another set of criticisms focuses on the tasks *Piaget* has employed to assess stage. A wide variety of studies have illustrated that multiple sources of variance contribute to performance on the common Piagetian tasks, many of these sources bearing little connection to logical competence. Thus, these tasks cannot be regarded as 'pure' measures of logical competence, in the way that *Piaget's* discussions of them might lead one to expect.

A final blow to the 'structured wholes' proposed by *Piaget* would appear to be struck by the criticisms that have appeared of the logico-mathematical models *Piaget* has used to represent them. Whether or not these models are conceptually incorrect or inconsistent, as some have argued, the few attempts to derive empirical predictions from them have produced negative findings. Overall, the models are sufficiently abstract and removed from measurable behavior that most observers would profess skepticism as to how such models would ever be validated.

The 'structured whole' debate, then, leads to the following fundamental question: Do developmental advances within individual domains occur more or less independently or, as *Piaget's* stage theory would demand, is there evidence of some form of 'unification' of these advances, across domains? In other words, do stages have any *psychological* reality? Do they exist from the perspective of the child, or only from the perspective of the theorist? If they do have psychological reality, what sorts of empirical data could serve as evidence of this? In the absence of satisfying answers to these questions, large numbers of developmental psychologists have turned away from stage theory, in search of what they see as more promising models in terms of which to conceptualize developmental phenomena.

Just at the right time, perhaps, coinciding with a growing disillusionment with *Piaget* and stage theory, another, seemingly very promising, alternative has appeared. Like the learning theory that developmental psychology relied on before *Piaget,* it comes from the mainstream of academic psychology, in particular the new thrust known as cognitive psychology, or cognitive science, that has taken hold there. The information-processing model has become popular very quickly in developmental psychology. This is so, perhaps, because on the surface at least, it appears to right exactly the things that many found wrong with *Piaget*. Where *Piaget* is abstract and metaphorical, it is concrete. Where *Piaget* is vague, it is precise and explicit. It seeks to explain performance rather than competence, process rather than structure.

Underpinning the information-processing model is the concept of the human as an 'information-processing machine with limited processing resources' [*Pascual-Leone,* 1980]. The model originates in the work of *Newell and Simon* [1972]. *Klahr and Wallace* [1976] made the first major attempt to apply it to developmental phenomena, in particular the concepts associated with *Piaget's* stage of concrete operations. The basic elements of the model are a collection of 'condition-action links' termed *productions*.

> 'The condition side of a production refers to the symbols in short-term memory (STM) that represent goals and knowledge elements existing in the system's momentary *knowledge state;* the action consists of transformations on STM including the generation, interruption, and satisfaction of goals, modification of existing elements, and addition of new ones' [*Klahr and Wallace,* 1976, p. 7].

Quite in contrast, then, to the study of 'condition-action' (or stimulus-response) links by behaviorists of the 1950s, the work of information-processing psychologists is focused squarely on modeling those processes inside the black box that behaviorists sought to bypass. An accepted test of the adequacy of those models is the test of sufficiency: The production system ought to be capable of producing the output behaviors in question. The techniques of computer simulation provide a ready means of evaluation in this regard.

A number of researchers have followed the general spirit of *Klahr and Wallace's* [1976] lead, though not relying explicitly on techniques of computer simulation. *Siegler* [1976, 1978, 1981], for example, characterizes children's behavior on Piagetian balance beam tasks in terms of several precisely defined 'rule systems' he hypothesizes the child uses to generate responses. The test of the adequacy of these rule systems is the extent to which a single rule system consistently predicts a child's behavior over a variety of balance problems.

Aside from *Klahr and Wallace* and *Siegler,* the two theorists who have been most closely identified with an information-processing approach to the study of development are *Pascual-Leone* and *Case*. Significantly, and this is a point we shall return to later, both *Pascual-Leone* and *Case* refer to their theories as 'neo-Piagetian', evidently regarding them as building on or refining *Piaget's* theory, rather than replacing it, as *Siegler* or *Klahr and Wallace* view their approaches. Others in the field, however, have tended to regard *Pascual-Leone's* and *Case's* work less as having any close ties to *Piaget's* theory and more as examples of the 'new wave' of information-processing approaches to cognition and cognitive development.

While it is less clear in *Pascual-Leone's* case, *Case* appears to subscribe to the central tenets of the information-processing model. He employs the more common terms 'strategy' and 'executive strategy' in place of *Klahr and Wallace's* 'productions', but the meaning is equivalent: 'Developmental structures are conceptualized as groups of executive strategies that can be modeled by computer simulation, rather than as logico-mathematical systems modeled by symbolic logic' [*Case*, 1978a, p. 65]. *Case* also talks about his theory, and in particular the ways in which it improves upon *Piaget,* in terms closely linked to the information-processing approach [*Case*, 1978a, b]. It is a *performance* theory, in that it is tied to the level of observable performance (rather than underlying structures or capacities). It is a *functional* theory, in that it addresses the processes producing that performance (rather than the structure underlying it).

Case, Pascual-Leone, and others, however, have criticized information-processing models on the grounds that they are unable to account for the occurrence of novelties. Accordingly, the claim is made, they are not genuinely *developmental* theories. Neither *Piaget's* logical structures, nor *Klahr and Wallace's* production systems, *Pascual-Leone* [1980] asserts, explain the child's acquisition of new strategies; in claiming to be the 'origins' of the child's strategies, they simply shift the burden of explanation to a deeper level (i.e. the origin of the 'origins').

Case [1978a, b] and *Pascual-Leone* [1970, 1980] propose respective versions of a theory they believe remedies this deficiency. (*Case's* and *Pascual-Leone's* formulations differ in a number of ways. The remaining discussion will be based on *Case's* version, since it has been published in a more explicit and complete form [*Case*, 1978a, b].) 'The general developmental factor', *Case* [1978a, p. 65] asserts, 'is conceptualized as a quantifiable level of working memory'. *Case* and *Pascual-Leone* cite research with a number of different measures of working memory, or M, that indicate regular increases in its size with age. They also describe a method of *task analysis* of psychological tasks with respect to their M demands. Knowledge of a subject's M power should then predict performance level on these tasks, and some empirical data are presented supporting this predictive power.

It would appear, then, that *Case* and *Pascual-Leone* have proposed a theory that incorporates all the advantages (of explicitness, precision, sufficiency, and so forth) characteristic of the information-processing model borrowed from mainstream cognitive psychology, while going on to propose an additional construct, M, that gives the theory a developmental dimension. This additional construct, they hope, can account for the developmental changes that must take place in a human information-processing system.

The Problem of the Missing Executive

In this section I shall undertake to express certain criticisms of the information-processing approach to development that I suspect will become well-articulated before the end of the present decade. As in the preceding section, I shall continue to focus on the particular formulation put forth by *Case*.

A critique of *Case's* formulation may seem premature. *Case* makes it clear in his presentations that he is still in the process of working out some of the fundamental propositions, as well as the details, of his theory; it is thus perhaps unfair to subject it to rigorous scrutiny, as opposed to appreciating its general thrust and intent, at this time. If we accept the view, however, that the limitations of any theory, or mode of inquiry, eventually reveal themselves [*White*, 1977], then the attempt to anticipate those limitations may make a contribution towards the overall forward movement of the field. It is in this vein that the present critique is attempted.

The critique centers on two issues, one more critical than the other. The less critical has to do with the method of task analysis. Task analysis, I predict, within a few years will be regarded as having less of the magical power that many developmental psychologists impute to it at the moment. In particular, it will come to be regarded as not very different in intent or strategy from what psychologists have always tried to do.

Case [1978b] spells out a procedure for performing a task analysis in more explicit terms than have other researchers who advocate the method. The first step he prescribes is to identify the goal of the task.

The second is to 'map out a series of steps by which a successful subject *might* reach this goal' (underlining mine). A recommended technique in this regard is introspection: Do the task yourself and list the steps you went through. Or, alternatively, one may use a purely rational method, plotting out a series of steps that would be logically necessary to solve the task. This analysis must be empirically checked against subjects' actual performance in a number of possible ways, e.g. confirmation that motor or eye movements conform to those that would be predicted by the theoretical analysis.

It is clear from this description that a task analysis is no more or less than a precise *hypothesis* about the internal mental processes that produce some observable behavior. As such, it must be supported by means of converging empirical evidence, using methods that have become traditional in psychological investigation. Moreover, it follows that there is no *one* correct task analysis of any given task. The potential for multiple hypotheses is comparable to what it is in any area of psychological inquiry; this is especially the case when one begins to formulate task analyses for incorrect or faulty task performances as well as correct ones, which is recognized as an important part of the enterprise.

One can hardly object to recent attempts by developmental researchers to analyze precisely the components that are entailed in a subject's solution of the familiar Piagetian tasks, more precisely than did *Piaget* himself. But the *intent* of such analyses is in fact identical to *Piaget's:* to understand the thought processes that underlie the child's behavior. To describe the 'strategy' or 'rule' the child uses to generate a solution was just what *Piaget* wished to do, though he did not employ that terminology. It is without question desirable that our models of the psychological processes underlying behavior become as precise, explicit, detailed, and complete as the state of the field will allow, and it is in the promotion of these characteristics that information-processing psychology has made perhaps its most important contribution. Developmentalists can easily appreciate the virtues of some of the recent analyses of Piagetian tasks, compared to the original analyses by *Piaget*. The formulation of such models in the first place, however, as a means of explaining behavior, has a history that goes back about as far as psychology itself. Modern 'task analysis', then, is an important endeavor, but it is not a magical key that unlocks the mystery of how a correct (or incorrect) performance is produced.

The second, and more critical, issue, with respect specifically now to *Case's* theoretical formulation, has to do with the M construct. It is my prediction that some such basic 'mental capacity' construct that increases developmentally will ultimately attain the appropriate empirical confirmation, though the measures developed by *Case* and *Pascual-Leone* clearly require a great deal of further refinement [*Flavell*, 1978]. I predict further, however, and this is the critical point, that this mental capacity will be recognized as a *necessary* condition for development, but not as a *sufficient* condition to explain how this development comes about.

Interestingly, there is some indication in *Case's* most recent writing that he is in fact moving towards seeing things in somewhat these terms: M-power may predict whether or not a new strategy will be acquired, but something else is needed to describe the process by means of which the strategy is acquired. *Case* recognizes, in other words, the distinction (which is often blurred) between factors that have an effect on a process (in this case, serving as a precondition for its occurrence) and those that comprise it. Recall that *Case* characterizes himself as a 'neo-Piagetian', and, quite interestingly, he resorts very explicitly to *Piaget,* in particular *Piaget's* mechanism of 'equilibration', in formulating his description of the developmental process. It will be instructive to take a close look at how he does this.

American developmentalists have not devoted much attention to *Piaget's* equilibration construct, focusing rather, as we have described, on the doctrine of stages. Equilibration has been regarded as the vague, rather mysterious, concept *Piaget* invokes to account for the transition from one stage to another. Given the vagueness of many of his stage characterizations, and the problems they give rise to, the tendency has been to regard *Piaget's* account of the transition between stages as a problem better postponed until the more basic issues of stage have been resolved.

In this historical light, *Case* [1978b] undertakes to recast *Piaget's* equilibration mechanism in what he believes to be the more productive information-processing framework; in so doing he promises to rid the concept of the vagueness and abstractness that has plagued it and transform it into an explicit, performance-linked construct:

'In the context of the new theory, the following general postulates may be assumed to characterize the sort of spontaneous conflict resolution that *Piaget* refers to as equilibration: (1) At any time when, in the course of some goal-directed activity, two pragmatically incompatible schemes are co-activated, the organism experiences cognitive conflict. (2) When the organism experiences such conflict, it temporarily abandons its current executive scheme and initiates a search for any other information that might help it resolve the conflict. In the language of computer simulation, one could say that it activates a heuristic executive scheme that directs a search of the problem situation, the problem given, and any stored information of relevance... (Postulates 3 through 5 refer to conditions that apply to this sequence of events, one having to do with M-power limitations on the number of schemes that can be simultaneously activated.) (6) If the conflict is not eliminated, the organism will, other things being equal, favor the response that is congruent with the greatest number of currently activated schemes. (7) After a very few trials in which the organism arrives at the resolution to its experienced conflict, the sequence of steps by which it did so becomes consolidated as a strategy, and the subject is able to generate the new solution on subsequent trials without the aid of any heuristic executive. In short, the organism forms a new executive routine for which the original problem situation is a releaser and for which the final solution constitutes the effector' [*Case*, 1978b, pp. 187, 188].

Case [1978b, p. 193] comments:

'... although perfectly consistent with *Piaget's* notion, the new characterization of equilibration permits a much finer grain of analysis – one that employs a much briefer time frame and one that can be tied much more closely to children's behavior in specific contexts... this characterization provides a link between classic developmental theory and current information processing theory.'

Case [1978b, pp. 194, 195] summarizes presentation of his theory thusly:

'To summarize, the theory originated by *Pascual-Leone* [and now developed by *Case*] introduces a number of refinements in traditional Piagetian theory, with the result that it becomes possible to identify the operational structures underlying performance on Piagetian tasks more easily and precisely and to specify the ... factors that affect the acquisition of these structures in greater detail. In most of its refinements, the new theory preserves the essential structure of traditional Piagetian theory.'

Is *Case* correct in his own assessment of his theory? Has he simply recast *Piaget's* account of the developmental process in more explicit, and thus potentially more useful, terms? I will argue that there is an important element missing in *Case's* formulation, seriously weakening it as an account of developmental change. The argument can best be made in the context of a concrete example. *Case* [1974, 1978b] undertakes a detailed task analysis for the 'control of variables' task. In the particular task, adapted from *Inhelder and Piaget* [1958], the subject must determine what variables (length, thickness, material, etc.) affect the flexibility of a set of rods.

The strategy for controlling variables, *Case* [1978b, p. 199] claims,

> '... is a relatively simple one ... All the subject must do is to identify an object with an extreme position value on the dimension to be tested (e.g. a long stick), then identify an object with an extreme negative value (e.g. a short stick), and then check to see if there is any *other* difference between these two objects that might affect the result of interest (e.g. bending).'

The M-demand of the task (the number of strategies that must be simultaneously activated) according to this analysis is three, leading to the prediction that children with M-power of three or greater (approximate CA of 7) will be able to master the task, whereas those with less M-power will not. *Case* [1978b] cites empirical data supporting this prediction.

Now it is certainly the case that the test just described (of the effect of rod length on flexibility) is not a difficult one to execute; one can imagine teaching 7- or 8-year-olds to conduct such tests without a great deal of difficulty. In this sense, we cannot quarrel with *Case's* assertion that the task is 'a relatively simple one'. I would contend that there is a more formidable challenge involved in this task, however, and it is attention to this aspect of the task that is missing in *Case's* formulation. *Case's* analysis is an analysis of a subject's ability to execute the sequence of strategies that lead to success on the task. There is another equally if not more important aspect of a subject's competence with respect to a psychological task, however, and that is the *knowledge that these are the appropriate strategies to apply,* in order to perform this task successfully.

What is involved in the case of the first aspect, or component, of competence typically is evident from the observable features of successful performance. What is involved in the case of the second component is less apparent on the surface. As in the control of variables case, it is often quite complex. It entails, for example, not just knowing what is right about the chosen sequence of strategies, i.e. being able to reflect on their value from a level one higher than that of the strategies themselves. Besides knowing what the chosen strategies 'buy one', so to speak, in terms of solution attainment and efficiency, such knowledge entails as well knowing what is wrong about every other potential strategy or set of strategies that might be applied to the problem – that they do not work (or work efficiently), why they do not work, and what mistakes they lead to.

In other words, I am making the distinction between executing a strategy and understanding the significance of it and arguing that it is the latter that may pose the more significant developmental challenge. In my own research related to isolation of variables reasoning [*Kuhn and Phelps*, 1982], for example, we have followed subjects over a period of months in repeated encounters with problems requiring isolation of variables reasoning for effective solution. All subjects began at a very low level of performance and showed a remarkable variety of wrong strategies in the course of, for some of them, eventually focusing on the right one. Their problem was not one of competence, with respect to possession of the relevant strategies, however; all of them exhibited the most advanced strategies on at least some occasions. There was a long period of vacillation, however, between valid and invalid strategies before subjects eventually stabilized their performance at the higher level. It was during this period, presumably, that they were developing some conviction about what it was that one needed to do to solve these problems effectively.

This distinction helps to illuminate why it is that M-power in *Case's* theory is a better predictor of whether a subject will be able to acquire a strategy through training than it is a predictor of the age at which that strategy is likely to be acquired during the natural course of development. Both conservation and isolation of variables, for example, have an M-demand of three according to *Case's* analysis, but the former normally appears a number of years earlier than the latter. Predicting natural age of attainment is at least as important, if not more so, than predicting teachability, especially for reasoning strategies, such as isolation of variables, that are not traditionally the subject of direct instruction. We can teach a child to execute controlled experiments, but will the child recognize that this is what needs to be done when an appropriate circumstance arises in the natural environment and no direct instruction occurs, i.e. most of the time? It is the second, rather than the first, aspect of competence distinguished above that determines the answer to this question.

Those acquainted with modern cognitive psychology will recognize a relation between this second component and the popular term 'executive' strategies. *Case* in fact makes reference to executive strategies in his own formulation, as one of three types of strategies he distinguishes. 'Operative' and 'figurative' strategies serve transformational and representative functions, respectively. 'Executive' strategies *Case* [1978b] defines as those that 'represent the series of operations a subject intends to execute'. This definition is ambiguous, however. It could refer either (1) to the operations (or strategies) themselves, or (2) to the knowledge that these are the appropriate operations or strategies to apply in this situation. In other words, it is ambiguous which of the two components of competence we have distinguished is being referred to. Accordingly, let us label the two possibilities executive-1 and executive-2 strategies, respectively.

After defining these three types of strategies, *Case* goes on to explain that the same 'unit' might serve any one of the three functions at different times or in different situations; in other words, the same strategy or set of strategies may serve an executive function in one context and an operative function in another. I infer from this that *Case* could not be defining executive strategies in the executive-2 sense and must have had an executive-1 meaning as his intent. (Part of the passage quoted earlier also supports this interpretation: 'In short, the organism forms a new executive routine for which the original problem situation is a releaser and for which the final solution constitutes the effector' [*Case*, 1978b, p. 188].) On this basis I have concluded that there is a missing executive (executive-2) in *Case's* formulation, and, as I've argued above, I believe the omission is an important one.

If I am correct in my assessment that executive-2 strategies are missing in *Case's* formulation, is this omission universal in developmental psychology or are there other bodies of research or theory that do attend to them? A likely source might be the rapidly growing literature on what has been dubbed 'metacognition'. This term has tended to be employed in a very general, often loose fashion. The two developmentalists most closely associated with the term, *Flavell* and *Brown*, offer these definitions: 'the voluntary control an individual has over his own cognitive processes' [*Brown and DeLoache*, 1978, p. 26] and '... one's knowledge concerning one's own cognitive processes and products or anything related to them' [*Flavell*, 1976, p. 232]. *Brown* [1979] acknowledges the generality of these definitions and notes that the current study of 'metacognitive' processes is not all that different from what used to get studied under the rubric of 'study skills'. *Flavell* [1979, p. 907], for instance, offers as an example of a metacognitive strategy the knowledge that '... one good way to learn and retain many bodies of information is to pay particular attention to the main points and try to repeat them to yourself in your own words'.

Despite its generality, however, at least some of what we wish to convey by the term executive-2 strategies would appear to come under the rubric of 'metacognition'. It is interesting to note, then, that *Flavell* parallels *Case* when he remarks on the interchangeability of cognitive (executive-1) and metacognitive (executive-2) strategies: 'Asking yourself questions about the chapter', *Flavell* [1979] says, 'might function either to improve your knowledge (a cognitive function) or to monitor it (a metacognitive function).' Thus, as becomes clear from his discussion, *Flavell* combines under the heading 'metacognition' the strategy itself (e.g. looking for the main points) and the knowledge that it is an appropriate or valuable strategy to employ in a given situation. I would not wish to be the one responsible for introducing a 'meta-meta' term into the field, and so I will stick with the executive-2 designation proposed earlier to refer to the latter. But my central point remains: It is of fundamental importance to differentiate one's knowledge of what one is doing from the knowledge of how to do it, and to devote appropriate attention to the former, as well as the latter. Current research in the field of developmental psychology, it is fair to say, has devoted comparatively little attention to the development of executive-2 strategies.

On the positive side, however, is the fact that a number of quite independent programs of research appear to have converged with respect to their conclusion that it is executive-2 strategies that should become the object of our research attention. That convergence itself is perhaps a heartening sign. Though neither is primarily developmental, two of the programs I have in mind are *Sternberg's* 'componential analysis' approach and Scandura's 'structural learning' approach [see *Sternberg, 1979, and Scandura, 1977,* for brief overviews of their respective research programs]. The objective of both approaches is to break down, in task-analysis fashion, a subject's performance on a psychological task into the individual units, or components, that comprise it. After considerable experience with their respective approaches, *Scandura* and *Sternberg* appear to have come to much the same conclusion: We can break down a task into its individual components and assure that the subject has mastery of each component; what is more difficult (and potentially more important) to understand is what makes the subject able (or, more often, what causes the subject to be unable) to assemble these components into a successful performance. Some 'executive' or 'control' mechanism, that governs this assemblage, both *Sternberg* [1979] and *Scandura* [1977] assert, is essential to an adequate theory of cognitive performance.

A third example comes directly from developmental psychology. Reviewing an extensive body of her own and others' work on the development of memory, *Brown* [1979] comes to a similar conclusion. Young children, she claims, often have in their repertoires the same basic strategies as older children and adults; it is primarily in the voluntary control of these strategies that subjects differ.

Piaget as Constructivist

How do executive-2 strategies develop, and how does this development relate to cognitive development as a whole? From the title of this section, the reader can guess that I am now going to propose that *Piaget's* work may offer some insight with respect to these questions and that his theory therefore ought not to be discarded by American developmental psychology. *Piaget's* work has been focused in a very fundamental way on the child's knowledge of what he or she is doing. It is reasonable to suppose, therefore, that he might have something to contribute regarding these questions.

I want to be very careful, however, to establish clearly the vein in which I would wish to make such an argument. I in no sense wish to serve as advocate or apologist for *Piaget*. That does not seem to be what the field needs most now. Nor is my purpose to lament how in focusing on the doctrine of stages discussed earlier American psychologists have 'misunderstood *Piaget*'. What a theory means must be viewed primarily from the perspective of those who are trying to make meaning out of it. The question of interest to me, therefore, is whether American developmental psychology can expand or alter its own conceptualization of *Piaget's* theory in a way that will be useful with respect to the most pressing questions it faces at the present time.

It is clear that *Piaget's* theory can be of any help with respect to the challenges and opportunities now facing American developmental psychology only to the extent that the theory is interpreted as about something other than stages. We reviewed earlier the conceptual and empirical dead ends the stage conceptualization has led to. What else, then, does *Piaget's* theory have to offer?

There is one virtue of *Piaget's* work that both advocates and detractors would agree on and that is that *Piaget* provides a rich, often fascinating *description* of developmental changes in the way the individual sees the world. The fact that young children do not regard quantities as invariant when they are perceptually rearranged, to rely on the most widely known example, now has abundant substantiation, and has fascinated millions who've heard or read about the phenomenon and perhaps observed it with their own eyes. And though the phenomenon has evidently been 'there to be seen' for centuries, no one noted it before *Piaget*.

At a minimum such phenomena are interesting, as attested to by the remarkable attention that has been afforded them, attention that goes well beyond any significance they may derive from their status as indicators of 'stage'. For the past several decades, American developmentalists of the whole range of theoretical persuasions have turned repeatedly to Piagetian tasks to elicit behaviors which they then subject to their own varied kinds of analyses. Why have American psychologists so frequently chosen *Piaget's* tasks as the object of their analyses? Are they for some reason uninventive in devising their own research tasks, or is it that *Piaget* was just particularly clever in discovering intriguing developmental phenomena?

While their intrinsic interest is not to be denied, there is something of deeper significance in *Piaget's* descriptions, and I think it is the at least implicit recognition of this significance that accounts for the fascination *Piaget's* descriptions have held for so many. And it is here, I would contend, that the key to a broader interpretation of his theory lies. Each of *Piaget's* descriptions of the young child's thought serves as testimony to the fact that the child is engaged in an extended 'meaning-making' endeavor, in other words is engaged in a *process* of constructing a conceptualization of self, other, and the world of objects. 'Childish' beliefs, like nonconservation, are of great significance for the fundamental reason that they cannot be a direct product of the external world, nor can they be preformed. In discounting these opposing alternatives, *Piaget* proposes at least the general form of a third solution: through a process of organism-environment, or subject-object, interchanges, the subject gradually constructs an understanding of both its own actions and the external world. This understanding is neither preformed nor imposed from without. The most important feature of this subject-object interchange is that it is bidirectional: the child and the external world must gradually come to 'fit' one another – neither makes any radical or unilateral accommodations to the other. Each new 'childish belief' that is discovered, i.e. each new belief that directly reflects neither the external world nor the child's innate disposition, provides further evidence of the occurrence of some such bidirectional interchange, and hence constructive process.

I shall assert at this point, and I am by no means the first person to do so, that it is the nature of this constructive process that is the heart of *Piaget's* theory. *Piaget's* fundamental claims regarding the nature of this process are at root just two. One is the idea that the process is directed toward adaptation, or progressively greater equilibrium, between individual and environment. The other is that the intellectual effort to understand one's own actions and their relation to the world of objects, i.e. the individual's extended 'meaning-making' enterprise, is a powerful motivator underlying this progress.

It is this constructive process, moreover, that is the foundation from which any doctrine of stages necessarily derives. In *Piaget's* investigations of the first 2 years of life [1952], structures and the construction process are never considered apart from one another. In his accounts of the remaining years of the child's development, it becomes progressively easier to separate descriptions of the structures themselves from a specification of the processes that gave rise to them. That American developmental psychology has assimilated *Piaget's* theory as a doctrine of structures, or stages, is probably an historical accident of its own position at the time it discovered *Piaget,* as we have discussed. But, in so doing, it has taken the theory out of the context of the much broader, and fundamentally more important, question of the nature of the interchange between subject and object. And it is *Piaget's* insight regarding this broader question, not his doctrine of stages, that stands to contribute to the future progress of American developmental psychology. The study of structures has come more or less to a dead end, precisely because one cannot study structures apart from or outside of the context of the construction process that gave rise to them. It is the process (of construction), not the product (the child's 'structure' or unique world view), that is most basic, and important. Indeed, structures can only be seen as temporal idealizations. If one wants to empirically test the psychological reality of stages, i.e. to investigate whether the 'elements' that comprise the hypothesized structure develop independently or whether there is some form of interdependence or unification in their evolution, one can only do so by studying the developmental *process,* for these alternative hypotheses are hypotheses about the nature of that process. Thus, even the study of stages becomes, in the end, a study of process.

As for the nature of the constructive process, and the subject-object interchange that comprises it, I would not want to argue that *Piaget* has provided an answer. I would argue only that he is asking the right question. Its importance is attested to perhaps by the fact that it is a very old question. It served, for example, as the focus of the entire intellectual career of the philosopher and psychologist, *James Mark Baldwin,* during the late 19th and early 20th century. *Baldwin,* an American, spent most of his career in American universities, but interestingly it was in Europe rather than America where his intellectual influence was felt. Though *Piaget* is often regarded in this country as without predecessor, the parallels between *Baldwin's* thinking and *Piaget's* are clear, and *Piaget* in fact made frequent reference to *Baldwin* in his early work. *Baldwin,* like the philosophers who influenced his own intellectual development, was concerned with the relation between mind and reality. How do mind and reality come to be coordinated with one another such that the mind can know reality as it is? The evolution of *Baldwin's* thinking about the problem is nicely described by *Wozniak* [1982], and is striking in its parallels with *Piaget:*

> '*Baldwin* was suddenly [following the birth of his daughter] confronted with the extreme cognitive immaturity and rapid intellectual development of the human infant. Clearly, the laws of thought could not be conceived to be as fixed and immutable as the laws of things. Reason, *Baldwin* was observing daily, is an evolving capacity of the human mind.
>
> The primary implication of this observation must have struck *Baldwin* with some force. The coordination of reason and reality could not be pre-established. On the contrary, such a coordination is a hard-won ontogenetic achievement. Over the course of individual intellectual growth, reason becomes progressively more adequate to reality. The coordinative epistemology must be conceived within a developmental framework. Yet, if the fundamental insights of the intuitional philosophy were not to be sacrificed, this framework must be constructed without retreat to pure empiricism. Developing reason and a stable material reality must be integrated in such a way that neither reason nor reality was lost. Thought, it was true, could no longer be conceived to be regulated by fixed native principles; but such principles must control the direction of intellectual development toward a progressively more adequate conception of material reality as it is. Reason and reality could no longer be conceived to be in pre-established coordination, but

this coordination, on which *Baldwin* had based his integration of metaphysics and science, must be the end-point toward which development is directed' [*Wozniak,* 1982].

If modern American developmental psychology discards *Piaget,* it is abandoning more than a doctrine of stages. In a word, it is abandoning the question of how the subject's evolving understanding of itself and the external world mediates the interchanges between them in a way that achieves their ultimate coordination. A case can be made that this is one of those fundamental questions that is worthy of continued asking.

On the Development of Theory

In this concluding section, I would like to return to *Case's* theorizing and the problem of the missing executive. In particular, I wish to address two questions. First, what is the significance of *Case's* omission of executive-2 strategies from his formulation, assuming my analysis is correct in this regard? Second, what insights does this analysis of *Case's* theory-making endeavor offer with respect to the enterprise of theory development in developmental psychology?

The 'neo-Piagetian' theories of *Case* and *Pascual-Leone* are particularly significant cases of theory development to examine because they attempt to build on and improve existing theory through a synthesis of previously unintegrated bodies of theory. *Pascual-Leone's* stated aim is to '... suggest how these approaches [Piagetian and information-processing] complement each other, thus correcting their respective deficiencies' [*Pascual-Leone,* 1980]. *'Properly modified',* he claims, 'information-processing psychology could well succeed in clarifying [*Piaget's* problems of stage and equilibration]' [1980, italics in original]. We saw, however, that *Case's* attempt to articulate an explicit formulation of this neo-Piagetian approach gets him into certain kinds of problems, and the problems he gets into are in fact very revealing.

Case recognizes that a capacity construct is not by itself sufficient to explain how development takes place. To formulate his description of the developmental process, as we saw, *Case* turns to *Piaget's* concept of equilibration: 'The child's attempt to introduce consistency or "equilibrium" into his cognitive system plays a major role in motivating his progress...' [*Case,* 1978a, p. 65]. *Case* makes it clear, however, that he wishes to recast *Piaget* while at the same time remaining faithful to the tenets of the information-processing model to which he subscribes. In taking on these dual objectives, *Case* embarked on a very difficult task, more difficult possibly than he realized. First, in adopting the information-processing model in which to cast his formulation, he may have bought more than he bargained for. In other words, he may not have fully appreciated the limitations that necessarily accompany the power of the model he chose. Second, he may not have fully appreciated the challenge of undertaking to integrate what are in effect two traditions that over a long period have shown themselves resistant to reconciliation.

It is more than an accident, I would hold, that *Case* failed to incorporate a dual executive, in the sense I have defined it, into his theory. The distinction between executive-1 and executive-2 strategies reflects a broader distinction having ancient origins in the history of psychology and philosophy. Can behavior (or behavior change) be adequately explained in terms of the causes that produced it? Or, for an adequate explanation, is it necessary to make reference to the intention or meaning of the behavior to the individual who performs it, i.e. the individual's *understanding* of what he or she is doing? This controversy between causal and intentional explanations of behavior is both an ancient and a modern one; *Dennett* [1978] presents some interesting new perspectives on it. It can be viewed, moreover, within the broader context of the long-standing conflict between philosophical traditions of materialism and idealism, and it invokes, certainly, fundamental and likewise long-standing questions regarding the definition of the science of psychology: Is psychology to be regarded as the psychology of behavior or the psychology of experience?

The reason, then, that executive-2 strategies are left out of *Case's* formulation is that *Case* is casting it within the framework of a model that is unable to incorporate them. Information-processing models of cognition, rooted as they are in the metaphor of the human as an information-processing computer, must of necessity come down on one side rather than the other of this debate. The information-processing model is committed to the causal rather than the intentional form of explanation precisely for the reason that, unlike humans, computers do not know what they are doing. Both the data it acquires and its own actions are of no 'interest' or meaning to the computer. Necessarily, the data are acquired out of the context of their meaning and the actions performed out of the context of their intention. The computer's lack of consciousness, or reflection, or volition, however, are exactly the characteristics that make its functions precisely specifiable and hence susceptible to reductionist analysis. It is exactly this dual set of features one is buying in adopting the computer metaphor.

It follows, on the other hand, that the information-processing model is not a particularly good one to capture the *meaning-making* (or executive-2) aspect of thinking or its development (and hence thinking as it occurs in its natural context). It happens to be just this aspect, however, that is essential to understand the Piagetian equilibration construct that *Case* wishes to encompass. 'The child's attempt to introduce consistency or "equilibrium" into his cognitive system', to use *Case's* [1978b] words, cannot be understood outside of the child's own meaning-making activity, i.e. the child's understanding of what he or she is doing. It is a psychological, or subjective, equilibrium toward which the organism is striving, not a mechanical one. It is within the framework of a subjective process of meaning-making, therefore, that the concept of equilibration must be understood.

If my analysis of *Case's* theory-making endeavor is at all correct, what lessons might be learned from it with respect to the development of theory in developmental psychology? Global theories operate essentially at the level of metaphor. Thus, we have the information-processing metaphor of the child as a computer, standing in contrast to *Piaget's* metaphor of the child as a philosopher or scientist, who directs the computer. Now, in some sense, we all recognize that both kinds of explanation are important. It is hard to imagine that we will ever completely understand a child tackling a difficult intellectual problem without a dual focus on the sets of executive-1 strategies the child brings to the problem and the executive-2 strategies by means of which the child coordinates his or her executive-1 strategies with the meaning attributed to the problem. Only through such successful coordination is a solution ever achieved.

Perhaps, then, what the analysis I have presented in this essay suggests is that we tend to take our metaphors too seriously. In a sense we function as slaves to the models and theories that currently dominate our field, working either as advocates to provide evidence to support the theory or as skeptics to provide evidence to discredit it, until such time as the theory is abandoned and the ties that bind us are released. *Case's* work is atypical in undertaking any theory synthesizing at all, but even he allows his enthusiasm for the power and promise of the new information-processing paradigm to blind him to its limitations and boundaries and thus to narrow his perspective on the problem he set out to address, in the end causing him to leave out what I have argued is the heart of one of the two theories he is attempting to synthesize.

However great our enslavement to theories may be, we are nevertheless quick to abandon old theories and approaches and to become absorbed with new ones. And ultimately a field makes progress through its succession of theories, for the excesses of any theory or research paradigm sooner or later reveal themselves [*White*, 1977], and in adopting and then discarding a theory one never goes back quite to the starting point. But my argument is, really, that there should be a better way to proceed. There are some enduring questions in psychology, certainly in developmental psychology, and we would do well to keep our eye on those questions and to see the theories that appear and disappear more within the historical context that these questions reflect. In developmental psychology, as I have attempted to highlight, these 'enduring questions' are particularly compelling: What are the mechanisms by means of which mind comes to coordinate with reality, by means of which the child becomes 'socialized' into the world of adults? *Case* recognized that it is essential for a theory of development to address mechanisms of change and turned to *Piaget's* equilibration mechanism as a basis for formulating his account of change. As we saw, however, he has handicapped himself by undertaking to work within the constraints of a model that is not well-suited to characterizing change, for the primary reason that it fails to incorporate the executive-2, or 'meaning-making', component of human thought that is almost certainly critical to its development.

Following a period of inital excitement over the powers of the new method of task analysis, even those developmental psychologists most committed to the new, information-processing paradigm as a replacement for all they found wrong with *Piaget* have declared the need to turn their attention to mechanisms of developmental change [*Siegler*, 1980]. This appears a heartening sign. The field of developmental psychology has been diverted for a number of years from its central question, the question of change, first by the preoccupation with *Piaget's* theory of stages and more recently by the enthusiasm generated by information-processing theory and task analysis as a substitute for *Pia-*

get. One wonders, however, will these researchers now go on to tackle this 'new' problem of developmental change entirely from within the perspective of their own current paradigm? Or will their inquiry benefit from the insight provided by a recognition of the larger historical context in which the question has been addressed, going back, at least, to *James Mark Baldwin?*

My thoughts focus in this regard not just on the established professionals who organize and carry out the field's work but perhaps even more on the generations of future researchers as they are introduced to the field during their graduate student careers. In particular, then, I think of the students of developmental psychology of the coming decades who may hear about *Piaget* only what was wrong with his theory and who may be introduced to the prevailing paradigm of the time as 'the way we do things', without gaining any appreciation of its historical context and thus of the choices that adoption of that paradigm reflects.

If we were to develop more of the historical sense that I have suggested, I would predict that theories in psychology would begin to appear and disappear less rapidly. It would become easier to find a theory is wrong in some non-trivial ways (and *Piaget's* theory stands as a most striking example in this regard), and yet to appreciate that the theory still has something important to offer. Furthermore, our exclusive focus on the testing of theories would be likely to decline, and we would begin to think more about how to refine and further develop our theories to address those questions that appear most important.

To argue against enslavement to our theories is not to diminish their importance. Quite the contrary, psychology has never been more in need of good theory. There are now signs of an 'ecological validity' methodology bandwagon that more and more researchers may be jumping aboard. When one ventures out into the real world to observe one's subjects, it is even more crucial to have a guiding conceptual framework to direct what one is looking for than it is in the laboratory, where method and question are more closely linked. Nor will the field outgrow its need for theory, as *Sears* [1975] appears to wish for in his assessment of the field:

> 'But scientific knowledge grows slowly, and when there is an absence of hard fact, traditional belief-systems become the guides to thought. The lacunae in knowledge are always filled with belief. Too bad that *science* cannot be divorced somehow from the

scientists, for it is they who have these confabulating systems that sometimes interfere with the objectivity sought through the precision of research' [*Sears,* 1975, pp. 59, 60, italics in original].

To the contrary, science is a construction by scientists, and it does not exist apart from the scientist's 'meaning-making' activity. A guiding assumption underlying this essay has been that we psychologists, like the developing child, gain in understanding from a metacognitive reflection on what it is that we are doing.

Summary

The present essay deals with the development of theory in the field of cognitive development over the last several decades. Particular attention is given to the rapid rise and then decline in the popularity of *Piaget's* theory and the current enthusiasm regarding the utilization of information-processing models. A focal point of the analysis is the 'neo-Piagetian' information-processing model proposed by *Case* [1978a, b]. There is a missing 'meaning-making' executive in *Case's* formulation, it is argued, and this omission is more than accidental. *Case's* work serves as an example of theory-making endeavors in developmental psychology, and the present analysis of his work is used to support a conclusion that we often allow enthusiasm for our theories to narrow our perspective undesirably. We would do better, it is argued, to remain more aware that there exist some enduring questions in psychology, particularly in developmental psychology, and to see the theories that appear and disappear more within the historical context that these questions reflect.

References

Brown, A.: Knowing when, where, and how to remember: a problem of metacognition; in Glaser, Advances in instructional psychology, vol. 1 (Erlbaum, Hillsdale 1979).
Brown, A.; DeLoache, J.: Skills, plans, and self-regulation; in Siegler, Children's thinking: What develops? (Erlbaum, Hillsdale 1978).
Case, R.: Structures and strictures: some functional limitations on the course of cognitive growth. Cognitive Psychol. *6:* 544–573 (1974).
Case, R.: Intellectual development from birth to adolescence: a neo-Piagetian interpretation; in Siegler, Children's thinking: What develops? (Erlbaum, Hillsdale 1978a).
Case, R.: Piaget and beyond: toward a developmentally based theory and technology of instruction; in Glaser, Advances in instructional psychology, vol. 1 (Erlbaum, Hillsdale 1978b).
Chestnut, R.: Television advertising and young children: Piaget reconsidered; in Martin, Current issues and research in advertising (University of Michigan Press, Ann Arbor 1979).

Dennett, D.: Brainstorms: philosophical essays on mind and psychology (Bradford Books, Montgomery 1978).
Flavell, J.: Metacognitive aspects of problem solving; in Resnick, The nature of intelligence (Erlbaum, Hillsdale 1976).
Flavell, J.: Cognitive development (Prentice-Hall, Englewood Cliffs 1977).
Flavell, J.: Comments; in Siegler, Children's thinking: What develops? (Erlbaum, Hillsdale 1978).
Flavell, J.: Metacognition and cognitive monitoring: a new area of cognitive-developmental inquiry. Special issue on psychology and children. Am. Psychol. *34:* 906–911 (1979).
Inhelder, B.; Piaget, J.: The growth of logical thinking from childhood to adolescence (Basic Books, New York 1958).
Klahr, D.; Wallace, J.: Cognitive development: an information processing view (Erlbaum, Hillsdale 1976).
Kuhn, D.; Phelps, E.: The development of problem-solving strategies; in Reese, Advances in child development and behavior, vol. 17 (Academic Press, New York 1982).
Martin, W.: Rediscovering the mind of the child. Merrill-Palmer Q. *6:* 67–76 (1959/60).
Newell, A.; Simon, H.: Human problem solving (Prentice-Hall, Englewood Cliffs 1972).
Pascual-Leone, J.: A mathematical model for the transition rule in Piaget's developmental stages. Acta psychol. *32:* 301–345 (1970).
Pascual-Leone, J.: Constructive problems for constructive theories: the current relevance of Piaget's work and a critique of information-processing simulation psychology; in Kluwe, Spada, Developmental models of thinking (Academic Press, New York 1980).
Piaget, J.: The origins of intelligence in children (International Universities Press, New York 1952).
Scandura, J.: Structural approach to instructional problems. Am. Psychol. *32:* 33–53 (1977).
Sears, R.: Your ancients revisited: a history of child development; in Hetherington, Review of child development research, vol. 5 (University of Chicago Press, Chicago 1975).
Senn, M.J.E.: Insights on the child development movement in the United States. Monogr. 40 (Society for Research in Child Development, Chicago 1975).
Siegler, R.: Three aspects of cognitive development. Cognitive Psychol. *4:* 481–520 (1976).
Siegler, R.: The origins of scientific reasoning; in Siegler, Children's thinking: What develops? (Erlbaum, Hillsdale 1978).
Siegler, R.: Recent trends in the study of cognitive development: variations on a task-analytic theme. Hum. Dev. *23:* 278–285 (1980).
Siegler, R.: Developmental sequences within and between concepts. Mongr. 46 (Society for Research in Child Development, Chicago 1981).
Sternberg, R.: The nature of mental abilities. Am. Psychol. *34:* 214–230 (1979).
White, S.: Social proof structures: the dialectic of method and theory in the work of psychology; in Datan, Reese, Life-span developmental psychology: dialectical perspectives on experimental research (Academic Press, New York 1977).
White, S.: Children in perspective: introduction. Special issue on psychology and children. Am. Psychol. *34:* 812–814 (1979).

Wozniak, R.: Metaphysics and science, reason and reality: The intellectual origins of genetic epistemology; in Broughton, Freeman-Moir, The cognitive-developmental psychology of James Mark Baldwin: Current theory and research in genetic epistemology (Ablex, Norwood 1982).

Wisdom and the Context of Knowledge: Knowing that One Doesn't Know

John A. Meacham

State University of New York at Buffalo, Buffalo, N.Y., USA

The purpose of this chapter is to explore, in a rather preliminary manner, the relationship between the constructs of intelligence and knowledge, on the one hand, and the social and historical contexts within which these constructs have been advanced and employed, on the other. This exploration is stimulated and guided by the view that human behavior can be understood only through the construction of interpretations which give meaning to that behavior. These interpretations at the same time come between ourselves, as social scientists, and that which we seek to understand. The significance of these interpretations derives not from their correspondence to a set of objective 'facts', but rather from their correspondence to the social and historical conditions within which they have been constructed. This is not the place to argue for this view – indeed, it is a premise for this book – and so the reader is kindly referred to more extensive presentations and discussions by *Broughton* [1981], *Gergen* [1980], *Habermas* [1971], *Meacham* [1978, 1981], and *Riegel* [1976a].

It would be inappropriate to define the constructs of intelligence and knowledge at the outset, since I intend to show that these constructs take on diverse meanings as they are considered within changing social and historical contexts. It should be apparent, however, that these constructs have occupied center stage within the discipline of developmental psychology, both conceptually and in terms of research efforts, for at least several decades. They are thus particularly important, and revealing, constructs to trace in any analysis of the development of developmental psychology, especially to the extent that they may illuminate the discipline's own knowledge-seeking activities.

The constructs of intelligence and knowledge are closely linked to the root metaphors of psychological theory, as well as to a variety of contemporary constructs such as memory, perception, problem-solving, and creativity. The validity of the construct of intelligence, however, has been increasingly questioned [*Samelson*, 1975], especially as this construct has been applied in the evaluation of women and minorities. *Riegel* [1973a] titled his introduction to a symposium on intelligence 'An epitaph for a paradigm', expressing the view that it was necessary to construct new, alternative conceptions of intelligence that were more appropriate for these and other groups in a changing society. The immediate stimulus for the present chapter, however, is the question of whether the traditional model of intelligence is adequate for understanding the course of intellectual development in adulthood and old age and, in particular, for capturing that quality of adult thought referred to as wisdom.

The chapter is divided into two major sections. In the first, a brief historical survey of changing conceptions of intelligence is provided, concluding with a critique of the traditional, accumulation model of intelligence. The main criticism – from the perspectives of the process of science and of intellectual developmental in adulthood and old age – is that the traditional model neglects uncertainties, doubts, and questions, and the role of social transactions in the construction of knowledge. In the second section, a definition of wisdom is advanced and illustrated. This definition is based on an alternative model of the growth and development of personal knowledge. This model is referred to as a knowledge-context model, in order to emphasize that the meaning and value of any knowledge depends upon the context within which that knowledge is known [*Jenkins*, 1974; *Pepper*, 1942]. The context includes not only other knowledge, but also gaps in the framework of knowledge. The knowledge-context model is consistent with recent emphases on metacognition [*Brown*, 1975], that is, the beliefs or knowledge held by individuals about their intellectual processes. Predictions from cognition or intelligence to personality and action may require an assessment of such personal beliefs, including, for example, beliefs regarding what is known relative to what is not yet known. The knowledge-context model provides an integration of life-span and cohort changes in intelligence, rigidity, cautiousness, and curiosity.

Intelligence in Social-Historical Context

Images of Man

I rely for the initial portion of this historical survey upon *Rosenthal's* [1971] remarkable book. His thesis is that broad and implicit images of human nature, and associated psychological theories and research, will reflect the ideology or spirit of each historical period, as well as the interests of dominant groups and classes within it. This thesis was explored by considering how a hypothetical psychologist, living in Classical Greece, the Middle Ages, or during the Italian Renaissance, might have conceived of and investigated intelligence, perception, group behavior, and the ego.

Rosenthal [1971] describes the Greek image in terms of the pursuit of excellence and truth and the striving for balance between diverse domains such as logic and emotion, intelligence and physical skills. Intelligence itself was viewed as multifaceted, including analytic intelligence, aesthetic intelligence, spiritual intelligence, political intelligence, and so forth. Overdevelopment of any one of these was to be avoided, in favor of a balanced integration of imagination, speculation, logic, and comprehension. The pursuit of intellectual truth for its own sake was encouraged and valued, including the questionning of assumptions, free speculation, imagination, and skepticism. The Greek concept of intelligence also included consideration of moral and humanistic concerns. *Rosenthal* suggests a variety of means by which a Greek psychologist or a contemporary psychologist might assess these diverse facets of intelligence, including asking persons to take a theme and develop it further, to compose incredible narratives, to find emotional aspects of logical material, and to analyze emotional experiences in a logical fashion.

In contrast, the image of man during the Middle Ages is one of concern with the symbolic and ritual aspects of daily life, rather than with practical affairs. The capacity to endure the frustrations, cruelties, and adverse conditions of life, while remaining virtuous and optimistic with respect to the promised afterlife, was taken as an indication of spiritual strength. A key intellectual ability was that of discerning symbolic or hidden meanings, through the interpretation of miracles, omens, revelation, and so forth. Empirical demonstrations were not as highly valued as subtle or clever logical proofs, nor were empirical demonstrations equal in force to authority as a source of knowledge. A medieval psychologist would have assessed intelligence with questions designed to measure symbolic imagination, subtleties of logical permutations, transposition of concrete issues into symbolic terms, and understanding of moral and spiritual themes. For example, persons might be presented with simple stories and evaluated on the extent to which they could recognize implicit moral issues, cosmic meaning, or spiritual significance in these stories.

The image of Renaissance man is one of uninhibited individualism, especially in the pursuit of rich and diverse aesthetic experiences and in literary and conversational activities. Although moral conventions were outwardly observed, it was understood that these could be covertly circumvented, and so craftiness, aggressiveness, deceptiveness, cunning, and so forth were highly valued. Of course, the Renaissance also represents a return to the classical ideals of unrestrained search for truth, as well as an increased emphasis on empirical observation and systematization of evidence. A Renaissance psychologist would have devised an intelligence test that assessed intrigue, artifice, social craft, cleverness, and ingenuity, as well as the capacity to optimize happiness and self-fulfillment. For example, persons might be asked to devise ways to deceive or discredit a fictitious enemy in order to gain a specified goal; to counter arguments during a debate with artfulness and ingenuity; or to demonstrate understanding of their own personal hierarchy of pleasure and self-actualization.

The Traditional Model

How can the current or traditional model of intelligence be characterized? *Sternberg* et al. [1981] provide one characterization, based on a factor analysis of ratings by laypersons and experts of behaviors of ideally intelligent persons. They found that both groups agreed on a general conception of intelligence that included a problem-solving factor, a verbal-ability factor, and a social-competence factor. This agreement is consistent with *Rosenthal's* [1971] view that psychologists not only study but also are influenced by and help to legitimize the currently dominant images of human nature. In order to move forward to a new model of intelligence, however, it is necessary to understand the relationship of the traditional model of intelligence to the social and historical context within which it has been advanced.

The ideal model for intelligent behavior has been the behavior of the scientist. The methods of science have their origin in part in the Renaissance, in the rediscovery of classical knowledge and the subsequent drive to add to that knowledge, to organize it, and eventually to achieve a complete and systematic understanding. This process of organizing knowledge was facilitated through the use of remembering systems, such as the method of places and images. *Yates* [1966] has argued that it was the elaboration of such systems, such as *Ramon Lull's* concentric circles, that made apparent the possibility of new relationships and of gaps in the organization of what was previously known. The goal of science, then, was to fill in these gaps and to attain a unified and encyclopedic understanding of all things through the accumulation of more and more knowledge.

Just as for earlier historical periods, there is a congruence between conceptions of intelligence and the dominant image of human nature; thus the model of the scientist as accumulating knowledge is consistent with a more general and implicit cultural image of accumulation. *Riegel* [1972, 1973a] has identified as one of the sources of this image the Anglo-American emphasis on competition in the accumulation of things, property, and wealth. *Looft* [1971] has argued that the belief in continued growth, and the belief that things are not good unless they are increasing, is fundamental to American life and also is reflected in the functioning of individuals and in contemporary psychology, which he labels a 'psychology of more'.

In psychology, this image of accumulation has been readily extended to encompass skills, habits, vocabulary, information, and so forth. *Brown* [1982, p. 107], reviewing the extent to which traditional learning theories, computer metaphors, and schema theories successfully address questions of growth and learning, comments that 'many current theories offer little more than an accretion mechanism'. Of course, on the European continent different social and economic conditions were consistent with the development of stage models of intellectual functioning, such as that of *Piaget* [1966]. Unfortunately, intellectual functioning in the stage of formal operations is typically interpreted in a fashion consistent with the images of the Renaissance mnemonist and of the scientist striving for an exhaustive arrangement of all possible knowledge [*Siegler and Liebert*, 1975; *Siegler* et al., 1973].

Critique of the Accumulation Model of Science

The accumulation model of intelligence must be criticized, however, for it does not accurately reflect characteristics of the process of science. Science is more than the accumulation and organization of 'facts'. It also includes the generation of uncertainties, doubts, and questions, and the loss and destruction of knowledge. Furthermore, science is not an individual enterprise, but rather a social activity. Both these characteristics will be discussed, from the perspective of science and from the perspective of intellectual development in adulthood and old age.

The role of uncertainties and doubts in the process of science is illustrated in the controversy surrounding laws recently enacted in the states of Arkansas and Louisiana, requiring that the story of creation be taught as a scientific theory in the public schools. Similar laws have been introduced in at least 18 state legislatures [*Hilts*, 1981]. The arguments for such laws are that controversy exists within the scientific community regarding the 'how' of the theory of evolution and that traditional scientific evidence can be reinterpreted to support the theory of creation. The American Civil Liberties Union and other groups, challenging these laws, argue that the theory of creation is not a scientific theory, but reflects instead a religious belief. The distinction between the scientific basis of these two theories rests on the fact that science is more than the accumulation of evidence (in the tradition of the Renaissance mnemonists); it also is the continual evaluation of that evidence in relation to what is thought to be known to this point in time. Thus, continued controversy over the precise mechanisms of evolution is consistent with the process of science; an unwavering commitment to a theory of creation is not. The distinction is neatly drawn by the anthropologist *Ashley Montagu*: 'Science has proofs without certainty. Creationists have certainty without any proofs' [cited in *Hilts*, 1981].

Montagu's distinction is reminiscent of *Gödel's* proof that the consistency of a formal system remains uncertain within that system itself and can only be established by reference to a higher-order system, which in turn will also lack certainty. Each successive attempt at a formal, consistent system will nevertheless retain an aspect of uncertainty and doubt, and for this reason no permanence can be attributed to the 'facts' or interpretations of science, all of which are potentially open to falsification. As *Bronowski* [1973, p. 353] has noted, 'There is no absolute knowledge. And those who claim it, whether they are scientists or dogmatists, open the door to tragedy. All information is imperfect. We have to treat it with humility'. While the traditional model of science emphasizes accumulation, it can now be seen that progress in scientific understanding is based also in the rejection of previous knowledge that is found to be incomplete, incorrect, inappropriate, and so forth. The loss or destruction of knowledge occurs simultaneously with the construction of new interpretations.

The traditional model of science also fails to give sufficient recognition to social activity as a defining characteristic of science. Scientific knowledge differs from other knowledge in not being derived from authority, as in the image of the Middle Ages, nor being constructed solely through the efforts of the individual, as in the image of the Renaissance. Instead, scientific knowledge is constructed through a process of social transaction [see *Meacham*, 1977, for a discussion of the concept of transaction], including exchange of ideas, criticism and debate, and agreement through consensus among peers in a scientific community. In describing the process of science, much attention has been given to the importance of methods of validation, including experimental design and empirical observation. These are certainly important in permitting falsification of hypotheses and in ruling out alternative explanations, and so decreasing uncertainty. But the major function of scientific methods is to facilitate communication among scientists, so that procedures, results, and conclusions may be clearly understood and replicated throughout the scientific community. The metaphor of accumulation is inadequate to describe the process of science, therefore, because scientific knowledge is not accumulated but rather is shared knowledge, both in its construction and in its application.

Critique of the Accumulation Model of Intellectual Development

These neglected characteristics of the process of science – uncertainty and social transactions – may also be considered as characteristics of intellectual development in adulthood and old age. The question of the nature of intellectual development during this period, including the existence of wisdom, becomes significant in the changing social context of increased life expectancy for increasing numbers of older people. In the United States, for example, the number of people over the age of 60 will increase by 16 million in the next 30 years, an increase of 50% over the current 32 million. These older people will be better educated and healthier and will expect a higher level of recreational opportunities and health and social services. Almost certainly there will be profound changes in how older people perceive themselves and in how society in general regards older people [*Meacham*, in press].

Those who study cognition in late adulthood and old age have shown considerable interest in identifying characteristics that are positive and healthy, that are typical of this age group, and that distinguish this group from younger groups. The concept of wisdom has received much speculative attention [*Clayton*, 1975]. *Erikson* [1950], for example, has described wisdom as an aspect of the successful resolution of the eighth psychosocial crisis in favor of ego integrity over despair. Many of the presumed characteristics of wisdom are similar to those suggested for a fifth stage of cognitive development, following the fourth stage of formal operations in *Piaget's* theory.

Both wisdom and the possible fifth stage appear to consist in part of an ability to recognize and to tolerate uncertainties, doubts, and contradictions and perhaps to make use of these in an imaginative and constructive manner to achieve an understanding qualitatively different from that of earlier stages [*Riegel*, 1973b]. *Labouvie-Vief* [1982] has proposed a post-formal operational, inter-systemic level of intellectual development, characterized by increased uncertainty (relative to an earlier intra-systemic level), as truth is discovered to be relative to the particular system within which it is validated. Other descriptions of the development of relativistic thought have been provided by *Perry* [1968] and by *Murphy and Gilligan* [1980].

These descriptions of uncertainty in thought do not make sufficiently clear the extent to which, in adulthood, a choice within a framework of alternatives implies a loss or rejection of previously chosen alternatives. In this respect, the first act of commitment in adolescence or young adulthood is easy, for one has only to choose from among the many possibilities of beliefs, values, identities, friends, and so forth. A second choice later in adulthood is far more difficult, for one must simultaneously and perhaps with considerable pain break with the beliefs, spouse, career, and so forth, to which the first commitment was made. There is increased interest in such second choices during the presumed transition of mid-life [*Levinson* et al., 1976]. Characterizations of this period of life include increased depression, as well as an increased ability to accept one's own tragedy as well as that of others [*Vaillant and McArthur*, 1972]. To summarize the present argument, these features of adult thought, including uncertainty, doubts, and contradictions, as well as the loss or rejection of beliefs, as intellectual development progresses, are neglected by the traditional, accumulation model.

The second criticism of the traditional model of intellectual development, parallel to the earlier criticism of the traditional model of science, is that the importance of social transactions in the construction of knowledge is neglected. *Sampson* [1977] has suggested that contemporary psychology has been too narrowly constrained by the image of self-contained individualism, so that psychological characteristics are conceived as located within individuals, to the neglect of conceptualizations in which these characteristics are viewed as the products of social transactions among individuals [who are themselves products of the transactions; see *Meacham*, 1977]. *Youniss* [1980] has provided an elaboration of this alternative view, arguing that social knowledge is not the product of private mental contemplation, but rather reflects cooperative dialogues among individuals of relatively equal status. It can be argued that the opportunities for such cooperative exchanges increase in adulthood, as the authority of parents recedes and as young adults find themselves engaged in work and community activities in roles of increased competence and responsibility. Further, the objects of knowledge in adulthood increasingly reflect social, moral, and ethical issues [*Levinson* et al., 1976; *Vaillant and McArthur*, 1972]. This social dimension of intellectual development in adulthood and old age will be taken up in the concluding section of the chapter.

The Knowledge-Context Model

To summarize the argument thus far, the accumulation models of science and of intellectual development in adulthood and old age neglect uncertainties, doubts, and contradictions in understanding, as well as the importance of social transactions in the construction of knowledge. At this point, an alternative model of science and intellectual development will be advanced and illustrated, one that incorporates uncertainties, doubts, and contradictions. The knowledge-context model is based on the relationships between only four concepts: K, all knowledge that the individual believes might be accumulated or acquired; k, that part of K that has been acquired and not lost; u, the remainder of K, representing uncertainties, doubts, questions, etc.; and p, the ratio of k to K. These concepts will be discussed in greater detail below. In addition, further points of contrast between the knowledge-context model and the traditional model of the growth of personal knowledge are described.

The Traditional Model

An implicit assumption of the traditional model of the growth of individual knowledge has been that there is a fixed, upper boundary on the knowledge that might be acquired (K). This boundary may be conceived differently according to various psychological theories or measurement procedures, for example, the set of items on an intelligence test, the content of a textbook or a professor's lectures for a semester, or all the books in a large library. The continuing accumulation of knowledge by an individual (k) is considered as progress towards the boundary. It is assumed that the boundary can be reached; that is, it is possible, although perhaps not likely, that everything there is to know can be known.

It can be argued, however, that there is no fixed boundary on what it is possible to know. *Fitzgerald* [1980] has noted that a basic dialectical contradiction in learning is that 'to know something is also to doubt it'. Although within the traditional model it is a contradiction to both know and not know at the same time, from a dialectical perspective such a contradiction is not problematic. The more one knows, the more one finds one does not know, and so learning and development necessarily continue. No doubt there is general agreement, even within the traditional model, that there is much that we can yet learn. What is startling in *Fitzgerald's* suggestion, however, is that, as the antithesis exists only in its relationship to the thesis, so the boundary of what may be known (K) *depends* upon what is already known (k).

From the perspective of the individual, the boundary on all possible knowledge is not permanent but rather is imaginable and continues to increase in relation to what is already known. Each new domain of knowledge appears simple from the distance of ignorance. The more we learn about a particular domain, the greater the number of uncertainties, doubts, questions, and complexities. Each new bit of knowledge serves as the thesis from which additional questions or antitheses arise. Consider as a rough analogy an individual living on a flat plain who desires to learn more about the surrounding countryside, and so begins to climb a mountain. The higher the individual climbs, the greater the area that can be surveyed and known and the greater the number of questions regarding additional features that might be seen by climbing even higher.

Within such a perspective, it is not sufficient to compare two individuals merely in terms of the objective amount that is known (k), for

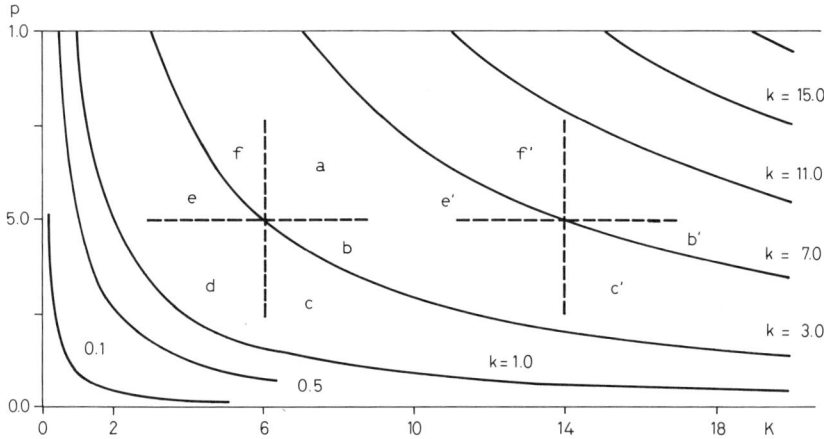

Fig. 1. Six types of movement within the knowledge-context matrix. K = Potential knowledge; k = acquired knowledge; p = ratio of k to K.

this amount has meaning only within the context of the potential knowledge (K) for each. For example, two individuals may appear to know the same objective amount, yet one may believe that he or she knows very little, while the other may believe that he or she knows a lot. In order to consider these complexities in the development of individual knowledge, it is necessary to consider simultaneously the continuing growth in potential knowledge (K), as well as the proportion (p = k/K) of potential knowledge that the individual has acquired (k).

The Knowledge-Context Model

The proposed knowledge-context model is represented in figure 1, a matrix determined jointly by one's perception of the extent of potential knowledge (K, on the abscissa) and by one's perception of the proportion or ratio (p, on the ordinate) of what one objectively knows (k) to all that can be known (K). This proportion may be interpreted as the confidence one has in knowing all potential knowledge. The amount of knowledge that an individual has currently acquired (k) may be expressed as the product of p and K. In this manner, gradients of equal k are described in figure 1. (Certainly the relationships between K, p, and k may be specified differently; k = pK has the virtues of simplicity as well as fitting the various examples set forth below.) An advantage to the knowledge-context model is that k, which is expressable in terms of the metacognitive or subjective variables p and K, may also be understood as similar to crystallized intelligence [*Horn*, 1970]. Thus, k serves as a link between the knowledge-context model and traditional models of the accumulation of personal knowledge. Uncertainties (u) are represented by the difference between K and k.

It may be helpful in understanding figure 1 to describe the perceptions of individuals located in various regions. An individual in the lower-left quadrant, for example, would know very little (k is small) but would also know that there is a great amount of additional knowledge that could be acquired (K - k = u is large). As a second example, two individuals in the upper-left and lower-right quadrants may have similar amounts of acquired knowledge (they may be on the same gradient of k). The first would feel quite knowledgeable; the second, however, would be aware of the great proportion of knowledge that had not yet been acquired. The latter would be more open-minded and eager to acquire more knowledge, yet possibly overly cautious in acting, due to excessive uncertainties.

Movements by individuals towards or away from various regions of the knowledge-context matrix have quite different characteristics. When both increases and decreases in K, p, and k are considered, there are six distinct directions of movement (fig. 1). These may be considered in detail, beginning with those for which K increases: (*a*). In movement of type *a*, p and k also increase. This common course of development, upwards and to the right, would yield the most rapid increase in k, because the distance between gradients of equal k is least when movement is perpendicular to any such gradient. Note that for each such increase in k, there is a simultaneous increase in K, reflecting the dialectical dependency suggested by *Fitzgerald* [1980], and in p, reflecting one's confidence in knowing a greater proportion of what can be known. An example would be the progressive elimination of each explanation in a series of explanations or hypotheses, such as suspects in a murder case. As each is eliminated on the basis of an alibi (k), new and more specific questions arise regarding the actions and motives of the remaining suspects (u increases, and so K increases). Since k increases proportionally more rapidly than K, one's confidence (p) in being able to solve the murder case also increases. Movement of type a is not without its dangers, however. As one approaches the upper limit of p = 1, one would have the feeling of knowing everything, even though the objective amount of acquired knowledge may remain quite small. Such an individual would be closed-minded, rigid, and lacking in curiosity.

(*b*) In the second type of movement, labeled *b*, p decreases while k increases. Movement occurs in this direction on the matrix when uncertainties, doubts, and questions arise faster than they can be resolved. This type of movement is illustrated by the experience of many scientists for whom initially small increases in knowledge (k) have had a substantial impact primarily because of the questions that were raised and subsequently pursued. Examples are *Freud's* conception of the unconscious and *Curie's* discovery of radioactivity. That a large number of questions can arise even following considerable increases in acquired knowledge was acknowledged by *Lashley* [1950, p. 477], in an article written towards the conclusion of his long research career: 'I sometimes feel, in reviewing the evidence on the localization of the memory trace, that the necessary conclusion is that learning just is not possible.' In scientific endeavors, one often underestimates the knowledge that must be acquired in order to answer a given question, for in pursuing the answer, more and more questions arise.

(*c*) In movement of type *c*, both p and k decrease. Some bit of knowledge previously acquired is lost (forgotten, or discovered to be wrong without the correct information being available), and the effect is to increase the range of possibilities (K). In *Christie's* [1976] *The Body in the Library*, the number of questions and potential suspects (K) is greatly increased when Miss Jane Marple concludes (k) that the body in the library has been incorrectly identified as that of the missing dance hostess. Not only must the body be identified, but also the dance hostess must be found.

There remain three distinct directions of movement for which K decreases: (*d*) Movement of type *d*, in which K, p, and k all decrease, may be illustrated by negative or regressive movements of type *a*. For example, entire domains of knowledge, including both the questions (u) and the answers (k), are forgotten. Suppose that for a particular individual, p = 1.0. It may be easier to move away from this state of rigidity by discarding a system of beliefs than by increasing the range of possibilities (types *b* or *c*). An analogy may be made with the shift from the Ptolemaic system to Copernican astronomy. Although over the long term the adoption of the Copernican system led to increases in both k and K, the short run may have seen decreases in both, as the Copernican system was simpler.

(*e*) In movement of type *e*, p increases and k decreases. This direction, in which the relative proportion one knows increases while both acquired (k) and potential knowledge (K) decrease, may be illustrated by the repression of a traumatic childhood event or by the belief system of bigotry, which depends upon blocking out both actual and potential knowledge regarding similarities between oneself and others. Entire domains of knowledge are excluded for the sake of the feeling of knowing well a smaller number of things.

(*f*) In the sixth type of movement, *f*, both p and k increase, while K decreases. In short, a potential area of knowledge is eliminated by the introduction of new information. For example, the surprise confession by the murderer eliminates the questions regarding the other suspects. Similarly, the failure by *James Cook* to sight land on voyages south of the Antarctic Circle in the 1770s brought an end to romantic notions of a rich and extensive *Terra australis nondam cognita*, the 'southern land not yet known'; and the journey of *John Fremont* through the western part of Nevada and the Sierra Nevada Mountains in the 1840s eliminated further search for the Rio Buenaventura, thought to flow westward from the Rockies to the Pacific [*Wilford*, 1981].

It would be preferable to be able to predict more precisely the relationship between changes in k and changes in K. However, the use that individuals may make of a given bit of information may vary considerably. One person may use the information to confirm existing beliefs (type *a*); for a second, the same information may lead to an expansion of uncertainties and questions (type *b*). The impact of an increase in k depends upon the knowledge context, as well as the individual's abilities to recognize and tolerate contradictions, to generate questions, to solve problems, etc. There is predictability only in the unique case of movement vertically. Here K remains constant, while k and p change together, and the knowledge-context model degenerates into the traditional model. This unique case may be illustrated by the memorization of a fixed amount of information that raises no questions, such as a list of letters, numbers, or words.

Development Across the Life Course

Can a general description of the development of individual knowledge over the life course be provided? In childhood, when k and

K are small, it is difficult to make gains in k (fig. 1, where the distance from k_n to k_{n+1} is large), but a small increment in k can result in rather large changes in K and p. It seems characteristic of childhood knowledge, not that the facts (k) are necessarily incorrect, but rather that they are understood in an immature context. Children are not well aware of what they do not know, and consequently new information is a great surprise and a source of wonder. Children also are often overconfident in the little bit of knowledge that they do have (p can easily be large).

As K increases, the range (in degrees) of movement of types *b* and *e* becomes less and of types *c* and *f* more (fig. 1, comparing *b* and *b'*, etc.). Movement of type *e* is an immature or regressive movement in the development of personal knowledge – one sacrifices both k and K for an increased feeling that one does know a lot. The range for this type of movement appears greatest when K is small, that is, for children.

With adolescence, and the acquisition of formal operations in thinking, the individual becomes able to construct all the possible alternatives in a given situation and to construct hypotheses contrary to known facts [*Elkind*, 1967]. This increase in the number of questions (u) corresponds to an increase in potential knowledge, K (type *b*). Questions increase for the adolescent more rapidly than they can be answered, and there is a danger of descending into what *Chandler* [1975] has termed epistemological loneliness, in which all points of view appear equally valid yet contradictory (p becomes very small). *Chandler* describes a range of regressive solutions to this crisis, involving the formation of systems of absolute and stereotyped beliefs (type *e*, opposite to *b*).

As k and K increase in adulthood, it becomes easier to acquire information (the distance k_n to k_{n+1} is now small). This change reflects the ease in acquiring additional information when there is already a good foundation of knowledge on which to build as well as a framework of questions (u) to guide the search for, and to facilitate the recognition of, appropriate information. An increment in k leads to smaller changes in p and K than for children (fig. 1), giving a greater stability to the personal knowledge of adults. For adults, new information usually is not surprising, but merely confirmatory, since it answers questions and fills gaps in a framework prepared to receive it.

In adulthood there is a lesser range of movement in the regressive direction *e'* and a greater range for *f'*. Direction *f'* may include some characteristics similar to those of e', that is, increased feelings that one knows a lot, although that knowledge is somewhat restricted, rigid, or stereotyped. In direction f', however, k continues to increase, and so this may be considered a more positive and mature direction than e'. Also in adulthood, there is a slightly greater range of movement in direction c', with a decrease in one's confidence (p) making one more cautious. There is evidence that older people are more cautious, refusing to act or make a commitment when refusal is an option [*Botwinick*, 1973, chap. 9].

No doubt the experience of older cohorts in recent decades is that the rate of expansion of K has been increasing, particularly in communication, transportation, medicine, values, etc. Except for those able and fortunate enough (in their careers or through continuing education) to learn about new areas of knowledge as rapidly as they appear (type a), a likely direction of movement is b: k increases, but not as rapidly as K, and so p decreases. One would expect older cohorts to become increasingly cautious, and this appears to be the case [*Botwinick*, 1973, chap. 9]. Another outcome is to move in direction f, leading to increased stereotyping and rigidity. Of course, in a traditional society, the rate of increase of K is very slow. In short, what is changing most dramatically for older cohorts is not k, the knowledge that individuals have, but rather K, the context within which that knowledge is experienced.

Wisdom

What, then, is wisdom? Throughout the life span, the easiest direction of movement is type a, which leads to high p, or confidence, with the consequent stereotyped closed-mindedness, lack of curiosity, and rigidity. The opposite extreme, for which p is low and cautiousness is excessive, is equally undesirable. The wisest course is to maintain a balance between the two extremes. The challenge of wisdom – to avoid the easy course of merely acquiring more and more knowledge – is to continually discover new uncertainties, doubts, and questions (u). The course of balance is roughly horizontal within the knowledge-context matrix, continually considering what one knows within the context of what one does not know. Only in this way can one give the appropriate consideration and value to what is known.

This definition of wisdom has been advanced previously, namely by *Socrates*, who sought to test the declaration of the oracle at Delphi that no one was wiser than *Socrates*. He questioned a man with a reputation for being knowledgeable and seeming to be wise both to others and to himself. *Plato* [1956, p. 427] reports *Socrates'* conclusion: 'I went away thinking to myself that I was wiser than this man; the fact is that neither of us knows anything beautiful and good, but he thinks he does know when he doesn't, and I don't know and don't think I do: so I am wiser than he is by only this trifle, that what I do not know I don't think I do.'

A number of suggestions for further research may be derived from this definition of wisdom: First, wise people should not be expected to differ from unwise people in the particular facts (k) that are known, and so research carried out within a traditional model, measuring only k, is unlikely to validate the concept of wisdom. As noted above, two people may have the same knowledge (k), but be at quite different points with respect to K and p. This statement seems an adequate description of the difference between a young and an old person, the latter of whom is wiser, by having taken a different route through the knowledge-context matrix of figure 1.

Second, wise people ought to differ from unwise people in their actions, that is, in the application of facts within a particular context that gives meaning to those facts. The decision to act is likely to depend to a considerable extent on p (or confidence) being high. Although high p may follow from movement of type *e*, oversimplifying or disregarding some of the complexities of a decision, a wise person would prefer to increase p through movement of type *a*. One behavior that may reveal such a preference is delay in making a decision, in order to provide time to actively seek new information or to discover alternative courses of action [*Meacham*, 1975, p. 165].

Third, wise people ought to excel at asking questions, for they have a greater insight into those areas of knowledge that they do not yet know about. The dialectical dependence of increases in uncertainties and potential knowledge upon what is already known implies that people ought to be more uncertain and questioning of topics with which they are very familiar than of topics with which they are only slightly familiar. *Iannotti* [pers. commun., 1979] has collected data from 80 college students, of whom 52 indicated that it was more difficult to evaluate themselves than an important person in their own lives (different from a 50–50 split at $p < 0.01$). Similarly, one would expect scientists to be better at discovering and creating key problems in their own disciplines than in others [but not necessarily better at solving them; see *Mackworth*, 1965, p. 53]. As *Getzels* [1979, p. 169] notes, 'a well-formulated problem is at once a result of knowledge, a stimulus to more knowledge, and is itself knowledge'. A related prediction is that wise persons, because of the questions they raise about their own knowledge, ought to be more cautious in making decisions based on that knowledge. *Reder and Anderson* [1980] have provided data consistent with this prediction, namely the more that was known about a particular topic, the slower were answers provided to specific questions on that topic.

Fourth, as *Socrates* did, the wise person ought to deny being and feeling wise, for the wise person appreciates how much he or she does not yet know. Data consistent with this prediction are provided by *Clayton and Birren* [1980]. Using a multidimensional scaling technique, they found older persons placed the stimulus word 'aged' farther from the stimulus 'wise' than did younger persons. This finding is unexpected in view of the common association of age and wisdom, but it is predicted by the knowledge-context model (if one assumes that wisdom increases with experience). This invokes the paradox noted by *Socrates*, that is, confession to being wise provides evidence that the person is not wise, while denial may be symptomatic of being wise. It is not surprising that the concept of wisdom has been elusive and has not yet been satisfactorily operationalized.

Fifth, in maintaining a wise balance between knowledge and doubt, movement in each of the six possible directions may be necessary. More particularly, one may become wise through a decrease in knowledge and/or an increase in uncertainties and doubts (types *c* and *d*). 'It is only when one recognizes one's relative ignorance and inexperience that one begins to question, to understand, and ultimately to grow' [*Lefkowitz*, 1979]. In being wise, it is not merely what one knows that is important, but also what one can admit to not knowing.

Conclusion

The knowledge-context model provides a framework within which such diverse constructs as intelligence, rigidity, cautiousness, and curiosity may be related and changes in individuals across the life span and between generations may be described. Knowledge in childhood or adolescence is difficult to acquire; it is also subject to wide fluctuations in feelings of the proportion of possible knowledge that is known and to the danger of regressive, stereotyped thinking. Knowledge in adulthood is easier to acquire and more stable, although slightly more open to the danger of excessive cautiousness. Wisdom is achieved by those who can maintain a balance between the extremes of rigidity and cautiousness, who can continue to acquire knowledge while simultaneously recognizing and constructing new uncertainties, doubts, and questions. A number of suggestions for future research have been proposed, as well as suggestions made as to why previous research on wisdom has not yielded decisive findings. Additional research questions include whether wisdom is associated with increasing experience or age and whether it is specific to particular knowledge areas or generalizable within individuals.

Apart from the concept of wisdom, the knowledge-context model contrasts with and calls into question several aspects of the traditional model of the growth of individual knowledge. First, acquired knowledge has meaning and value to the individual only in the *context* of what else is known and not known. Within the traditional model, it has been assumed that each particular fact has equivalent importance across individuals (e.g. items on tests). Second, within the knowledge-context model an important factor in the prediction of personality and action may be metacognitive processes, including the individual's perception of how much he or she knows and does not know. In contrast, within the traditional model it has been assumed that direct relationships between the knowledge of individuals (e.g. scores on tests) and personality and action could be verified.

Third, within the knowledge-context model it is not possible to set limits or boundaries on what may be known. The accumulation of knowledge by the individual is instrumental in changing the individual's perception of the uncertainties, doubts, and questions remaining to be resolved. The activity of knowing brings about the conditions under which further knowing, change, and development will necessarily occur. As *Riegel* [1976 b, p. 697] notes, 'developmental and historical tasks are never completed. At the very moment when completion seems to be achieved, new questions and doubts arise in the individual and society'. Similarly, in *Piaget's* equilibration model of development,

'While perturbations are integrated and the system reorganized, new gaps and contradictions occur. Metaphorically speaking, reality backs up while it is approached by the subject who tries to understand it. There is an infinite regression of gaps and perturbations in the growth of knowledge. A given perturbation may be temporary, but the existence of perturbations seems essential to the growing of knowledge. It is important to note that ignorance and knowledge grow together, just as reorganization and perturbations do' [*Moessinger*, 1978, p. 263].

This perspective may be contrasted with learning theory or information-processing approaches, for example, in which knowledge becomes more complete with experience, and the proportion that one does not know becomes less.

Fourth, the development of personal knowledge cannot be adequately described, and individuals and groups (such as the young and the old) cannot be compared to one another, by reference to increases and decreases along a single dimension. In particular, wisdom is not defined as more of a particular quality, but rather as a balance between qualities (cf. the Greek image of human nature). The knowledge-context model allows for a multitude of developmental routes and states of personal knowledge and directs attention to the assessment not merely of how much is known (k), but also of changes in the confidence with which that knowledge is held (p) and in the frequency and sophistication with which questions are raised (u and K). These latter changes provide the opportunity for future growth of personal knowledge.

Many preschool programs, and indeed liberal education, define as goals not merely the acquisition of specific information but also the development of abilities to raise questions and critically evaluate current knowledge, to apply knowledge to achieve desired goals, and to make original and creative contributions to existing knowledge. Unfortunately, much controversy over the success of innovative educational programs may reflect the evaluation of these programs only within the traditional model emphasizing the single dimension of accumulation of knowledge (k), rather than along a variety of dimensions derived from the educational goals of the program. For example, an educational program intended to raise questions and thus stimulate increases in perceptions of potential knowledge (K; type *c*) may show short-term decreases in the acquired knowledge (k) of the students, or apparent regression, if evaluated only by the single criterion of the traditional model.

Fifth, I must return to the neglect in traditional models of intelligence of the role of social transactions, a neglect that has apparently not been rectified within the proposed knowledge-context model. If one asks, however, under what conditions uncertainties, doubts, and questions are most likely to arise, and thus to prepare the way for further intellectual development, the answer must be that they arise in social transactions, in dialogue which provides the means for the construction of new knowledge. This emphasis on social transactions is entirely consistent with *Piaget's* model of equilibration, as presented by *Furth* [1981], in which 'the sharing of knowledge with others is an intrinsic part of having knowledge, and cooperation and dialogue are the primary occasions that set the stage for increasing knowledge' [see also *Youniss*, this volume, for an elaboration of this view].

If the development of developmental psychology is evaluated in terms of the traditional, accumulation model of science, then one might have cause for despair. Certainly in recent decades there has been an accumulation of graduate programs, of developmental researchers, of more sophisticated research methods, and of articles and books on human development. It is less certain, however, that there has been an accumulation of useful knowledge about changes in social and psychological processes across the life course. Concepts and 'facts' that were considered basic to the discipline only a few years ago are now rarely mentioned. Yet this is altogether reasonable within the framework of the knowledge-context model. The introduction of new knowledge changes the broader context within which all knowledge is evaluated, and so the evaluation of knowledge and the construction of new interpretations must always be a continuing process. The development of developmental psychology may thus be characterized not merely as an accumulative movement of type *a*, but rather as a combination of all the various types of movement. Our discipline can remain healthy and progressive as long as we maintain a balance between confidence in what is known and doubts regarding what is not yet known, and as long as we continue to construct new interpretations of the course of human development that are appropriate to contemporary social and historical contexts [*Meacham*, 1981].

Summary

This chapter concerns two constructs that have played a central role in the thinking and research activities of developmental psychologists, the constructs of intelligence and knowledge. The purpose of the chapter is to explore, in a rather preliminary manner, the relationship between these constructs, on the one hand, and the social and historical contexts in which these constructs have developed, on the other. A brief historical survey of changing conceptions of intelligence is provided, concluding with a critique of the traditional, accumulation model. The main criticism – from the dual perspectives of the process of science and intellectual development in adulthood and old age – is that the traditional model neglects uncertainties, doubts, and questions, as well as the role of social transactions in the construction of knowledge. An alternative, knowledge-context model is advanced and illustrated, within which wisdom is defined as a balance between increases in the amount that one knows and simultaneous increases in the recognition that there is much that one does not know. As well as providing an integration of life-span and cohort changes in intelligence, rigidity, cautiousness, and curiosity, it is claimed, the knowledge-context model offers a more accurate and fruitful way of conceptualizing knowledge development both in science and within the individual.

Acknowledgements

The author wishes to thank *Eleanor A. Jacobs* for her advice and encouragement. An earlier version of the knowledge-context model was presented at the Institute for Life-Span Development and Gerontology, University of Akron, February 1980, and at the meeting of the International Society for the Study of Behavioral Development, Toronto, August 1981.

References

Botwinick, J.: Aging and behavior (Springer, New York 1973).
Bronowski, J.: The ascent of man (Little, Brown, Boston 1973).
Broughton, J.M.: Piaget's structural developmental theory. V. Ideology-critique and the possibility of a critical developmental theory. Hum. Dev. *24:* 382–411 (1981).
Brown, A.L.: The development of memory: knowing, knowing about knowing, and knowing how to know; in Reese, Advances in child development and behavior, vol. 10 (Academic Press, New York 1975).
Brown, A.L.: Learning and development: the problems of compatibility, access, and induction. Hum. Dev. *25:* 89–115 (1982).
Chandler, M.J.: Relativism and the problem of epistemological loneliness. Hum. Dev. *18:* 171–180 (1975).
Christie, A.: The body in the library (Pocket, New York 1976).
Clayton, V.: Erikson's theory of human development as it applies to the aged: wisdom as contradictive cognition. Hum. Dev. *188:* 119–128 (1975).
Clayton, V.P.; Birren, J.E.: The development of wisdom across the life span: a re-examination of an ancient topic; in Baltes, Brim, Life-span development and behavior, vol. 3 (Academic Press, New York 1980).
Elkind, D.: Egocentrism in adolescence. Child Dev. *38:* 1025–1034 (1967).
Erikson, E.H.: Childhood and society (Norton, New York 1950).

Fitzgerald, J.M.: Learning and development: mutual bases in a dialectical perspective. Hum. Dev. 23: 376-382 (1980).
Furth, H.G.: Piaget's new equilibration model; in Furth, Piaget and knowledge; 2nd ed. (University of Chicago Press, Chicago 1981).
Gergen, K.J.: The emerging crisis in life-span developmental theory; in Baltes, Brim, Life-span development and behavior, vol. 3 (Academic Press, New York 1980).
Getzels, J.W.: Problem finding: a theoretical note. Cognitive Sci. 3: 167-172 (1979).
Habermas, J.: Knowledge and human interests (Beacon Press, Boston 1971).
Hilts, P.J.: 'Creationism' back in schools as new science. The Washington Post, July 23, 1981, p. Al.
Horn, J.L.: Organization of data on life-span development of human abilities; in Goulet, Baltes, Life-span developmental psychology: Research and theory (Academic Press, New York 1970).
Jenkins, J.J.: Remember that old theory of memory? Well, forget it! Am. Psychol. 29: 785-795 (1974).
Labouvie-Vief, G.: Dynamic development and mature autonomy: a theoretical prologue. Hum. Dev. 25: 161-191 (1982).
Lashley, K.S.: In search of the engram. Symp. Soc. exp. Biol. 4: 454-482 (1950).
Lefkowitz, M.R.: Education for women in a man's world. Chronicle of Higher Education, August 6, 1979, p. 56.
Levinson, D.J.; Darrow, C.M.; Klein, E.B.; Levinson, M.H.; McKee, B.: Periods in the adult development of men: ages 18 to 45. Counsel. Psychol. 6: 21-25 (1976).
Looft, W.R.: The psychology of more. Am. Psychol. 26: 561-565 (1971).
Mackworth, N.H.: Originality. Am. Psychol. 20: 51-66 (1965).
Meacham, J.A.: A dialectical approach to moral judgment and self-esteem. Hum. Dev. 18: 159-170 (1975).
Meacham, J.A.: A transactional model of remembering; in Datan, Reese, Life-span developmental psychology: dialectical perspectives on experimental research (Academic Press, New York 1977).
Meacham, J.A.: History and developmental psychology. Hum. Dev. 218: 363-369 (1978).
Meacham, J.A.: Political values, conceptual models, and research; in Lerner, Busch-Rossnagel, Individuals as producers of their development (Academic Press, New York 1981).
Meacham, J.A.: Aging, work, and youth: new words for a new age of old age; in Bain, The sociogenesis of language and human conduct (Plenum Press, New York, in press).
Moessinger, P.: Piaget on contradiction. Hum. Dev. 218: 255-267 (1978).
Murphy, J.M.; Gilligan, C.: Moral development in late adolescence and adulthood: a critique and reconstruction of Kohlberg's theory. Hum. Dev. 23: 77-104 (1980).
Pepper, S.C.: World hypotheses (University of California Press, Berkeley 1942).
Perry, W.G.: Forms of intellectual and ethical development in the college years (Holt, Rinehart & Winston, New York 1968).
Piaget, J.: Psychology of intelligence (Littlefield, Adams, Totawa 1966).
Plato: The apology (The defense of Socrates); in Rouse (trans.), Great dialogues of Plato, (Mentor, New York 1956).
Reder, L.M.; Anderson, J.R.: A partial resolution of the paradox of interference: the role of integrating knowledge. Cognitive Psychol. 12: 447-472 (1980).

Riegel, K.F.: The influence of economic and political ideologies upon the development of developmental psychology. Psychol. Bull. *78:* 129-144 (1972).

Riegel, K.F.: An epitaph for a paradigm: introduction for a symposium. Hum. Dev. *16:* 1-7 (1973); also in Riegel, Intelligence: alternative views of a paradigm (Karger, Basel 1973a).

Riegel, K.F.: Dialectical operations: the final period of cognitive development. Hum. Dev. *16:* 346-370 (1973b).

Riegel, K.F.: Psychology of development and history (Plenum, New York 1976a).

Riegel, K.F.: The dialectics of human development. Am. Psychol. *31:* 689-700 (1976b).

Rosenthal, B.G.: The images of man (Basic Books, New York 1971).

Samelson, F.: On the science and politics of IQ. Soc. Res. *42:* 467-488 (1975).

Sampson, E.E.: Psychology and the American ideal. J. Personal. soc. Psychol. *35:* 767-782 (1977).

Siegler, R.S.; Liebert, R.M.: Acquisition of formal scientific reasoning by 10- and 13-year-olds: designing a factorial experiment. Devl. Psychol. *11:* 401-402 (1975).

Siegler, R.S.; Liebert, D.E.; Liebert, R.M.: Inhelder and Piaget's pendulum problem: teaching preadolescents to act as scientists. Devl. Psychol. *9:* 97-101 (1973).

Sternberg, R.J.; Conway, B.E.; Ketron, J.L.; Bernstein, M.: People's conceptions of intelligence. J. Personal. soc. Psychol. *41:* 37-55 (1981).

Vaillant, G.E.; McArthur, C.C.: Natural history of male psychologic health. I. The adult life cycle from 18-50. Semin. Psychiat. *4:* 415-427 (1972).

Wilford, J.N.: The mapmakers (Knopf, New York 1981).

Yates, F.A.: The art of memory (University of Chicago Press, Chicago 1966).

Youniss, J.: Parents and peers in social development (University of Chicago Press, Chicago 1980).

Cultural Practices and Piagetian Theory: The Impact of a Cross-Cultural Research Program

Denis Newman, Margaret Riel, Laura M.W. Martin

University of California at San Diego, La Jolla, Calif., USA

When the United Nations adopted the Universal Declaration of Human Rights in 1948, *Piaget* [1973] wrote a commentary on the article which stated that every person has the right to education. The central thesis of *Piaget's* [1973] commentary is that education should not attempt to coerce the younger generation into believing a particular set of commonly accepted truths. Rather, education must be directed to the personality, which requires free and spontaneous activity based on collaboration rather than submissiveness. For *Piaget*, cognitive development is a universal process that goes on independent of culture-specific teaching and even *in spite of* educational practices that are directed toward conformity and collective standards.

The cross-cultural arena, then, is a seemingly appropriate place to test *Piaget's* theory. In 1948, when *Piaget* published his commentary, there had been little research outside of Western cultures to ascertain whether or not the type of process described by *Piaget* did in fact operate universally. Over the last few decades, a large body of cross-cultural research has been accumulated [*Dasen and Heron*, 1981]. In this chapter, we examine the implications of recent cross-cultural research for *Piaget's* theory and its underlying assumptions about the relation between cognition and culture.

Piaget's Program for Cross-Cultural Research

Along with the growing interest in *Piaget's* theory among developmental psychologists during the 1960's came an interest in using his tasks as tools for cross-cultural comparisons. The early results of psychologists returning from the field were not clearly favorable to his theory. *Piaget's* central thesis is that the process by which the child constructs or invents logical knowledge, equilibration, is a product of the child's interaction with the environment. Formal education, then, should not be a necessary condition for cognitive development. But *Greenfield* [1966], returning from Senegal, suggested that for the children she studied, 'without school, intellectual development, defined as *any* qualitative change, ceases shortly after age nine'[p. 234].

In response to evidence from non-Western cultures, *Piaget* [1974] attempted to clarify the theoretical issues at stake by outlining a program of cross-cultural research. He wanted to use cross-cultural evidence to help decide among three competing hypotheses concerning the process of cognitive development: (1) a biological maturational process is sufficient for cognitive development; (2) the equilibration process accounts for cognitive development; (3) a process of specific educational transmission is necessary for cognitive development.

Each of the three hypotheses predicted a different relation between a set of independent and dependent variables. The independent variables are the features of the culture that, in theory, influence the rate and/or end point of development. The dependent variables are the rate and end point of cognitive development as measured by the tasks *Piaget* used in his own research. Each hypothesized process (i.e. maturation, equilibration or education) could be considered as mediating between the outcome (rate and end point of development) and the environmental variables that influence it. The pattern of relations between the environmental factors and rate and end point of development might then be used to confirm one of the competing hypotheses (or at least disconfirm the others).

As *Piaget* [1974] expressed it, there were four 'factors' that had to be considered. Each of these factors is associated with one of the three hypotheses and with features of the cultural environment that would be expected to influence cognitive development if that hypothesis were correct. While there are four factors, there are only three hypotheses. This is because the equilibration process can be influenced by features of both the social and non-social environment.

1. Biological Factors. These are presumably the same for all cultures. If the biological hypothesis is correct, *Piaget* would expect little or no effect of sociocultural environment on either the developmental sequence that unfolds or on the rate at which the unfolding occurs.

2. Equilibration Factors. These factors have to do with the child's general activity and interaction with the environment. *Piaget* assumes that the child can construct logical structures on the basis of interactions with those aspects of the physical environment that are so general that they are present in *any* culture. If the equilibration hypothesis is correct, then the same developmental sequence should occur regardless of the specific features of the culture. But cultures may differ in the extent to which their particular practices provide chances to explore and experiment freely with the environment, or what Piagetians call 'operatory exercise'. To the extent that such variations exist, *Piaget* predicts that different cultures will retard or accelerate the equilibration process and hence the rate of development. Since such differences in the cultural environment would not affect a purely maturational process, finding differences in the rate of development related to these cultural differences would rule out maturational processes as the primary determinant of cognitive development.

3. Social Factors of Interpersonal Coordination. While the first two factors are concerned with the effects of the *individual's* biology and activity, the second two factors are concerned with the effects of the social environment. *Piaget* distinguishes between effects of the teachings of a particular culture (factor 4) and effects of features that all societies have in common (factor 3). *Piaget* [1974, p. 302] notes that 'in any environment individuals ask questions, exchange information, work together, argue, object, etc.' According to his theory, these exchanges create an equilibration process operating at the inter-individual level of social relations, just as the coordination of an individual's actions results from an equilibration process operating within the individual. Thus, if the equilibration hypothesis is correct, cultural differences in opportunities to interact with others should have as profound an effect on the rate of development as differences in opportunities for the individual to explore the environment (factor 2). Accordingly, *Piaget* expects a faster rate of development in cultures providing a high level of such opportunities. As with factor 2, however, he would not expect these cultural differences to affect the sequence of development.

4. Factors of Educational and Cultural Transmission. The final factor includes all the specific features that make the social environment of one culture different from that of another. If research were to show that the sequence of logical structures exists in some but not all cultures, specific cultural transmission would be implicated as a critical factor in the developmental process. It would also follow that the critical experiences necessary for development are not as general as *Piaget* supposed.

The four factors *Piaget* outlined are confounded in any single culture. Like that of most cross-cultural research programs, the concern of *Piaget's* program is to dissociate these factors. He illustrates the need to unconfound the factors with a study by *Mosheni* [1966] that compared urban and rural children in Iran. A delay of 2-3 years in mastery of concrete operational tasks was found among the rural children, while those in Teheran performed roughly as those in Geneva. *Piaget* [1974; pp. 305, 306] notes, however, that with the exception of biological factors, it is not possible to specify which of his factors should be implicated in the Iranian rural-urban contrast:

> 'Concerning factor 2, *Mosheni* noticed the astounding lack of activity of the young country children who do not go to school and who have no toys, except stones or sticks, and who show a constant passivity and apathy. Thus, one finds at the same time a poor development of the coordinations of individual actions (factor 2), of interpersonal actions (factor 3), and educational transmissions (factor 4), which are reduced since these children are illiterate. This implies a convergence of the three groups of factors.'

Piaget thus calls for further studies in which each factor is more clearly controlled. This research could be accomplished by comparing cultures that differ with respect to just one of the factors.

Though *Piaget* is usually considered a universalist, in important respects he needed cultural *differences* in order to make the necessary dissociation possible. Qualitative differences in the content of what different cultures taught their young would not be sufficient. *Piaget* needed also to identify quantitative differences in the opportunities provided for children to interact with a physical (factor 2) and social (factor 3) environment, regardless of the specific content of those interactions, because he predicted these differences would have an impact on the rate at which the equilibration process occurred. Without substantial cultural differences of these types, it would be impossible to dissociate equilibration factors from factors of educational transmission.

In the discussion that follows, we observe that carrying out this cross-cultural research program has not been easy. There has been considerable discussion of the methodological problems involved in attempting to measure development in other cultures using *Piaget's* tasks. Without denying the importance of the problem of assessing development in other cultures, we will focus our discussion primarily on another kind of problem that has generally received less attention. This is the problem of identifying and measuring the environmental characteristics that are hypothesized to influence development. It is this aspect of the cross-cultural research enterprise that most clearly involves *Piaget's* central assumptions about the relation of culture and thought. In particular, *Piaget* assumes that cultures can be characterized in terms of the opportunities they provide for operatory exercise independently of their specific cultural practices. Cross-cultural research has found, however, a close relation between specific practices and levels of development, suggesting the need to question the independence of factors 2 and 3 from factor 4.

Evidence for Cultural Variability

The number of studies using Piagetian tasks in non-Western cultures is extensive [see Dasen and Heron, 1981, for a recent review]. Most of these studies have used 'concrete operational' tasks. This is so perhaps because the concrete operational stage of logical development usually appears in Western cultures during the first few years of schooling and so has special significance for the issue of schooling effects. A smaller number of studies has examined the more advanced formal operational tasks. Typically, several age groups are sampled and the age at which given percentages of the various groups 'pass' the test are compared to one another and to age norms from the studies conducted in Geneva (or in other cultures of interest).

The pattern of results has not changed radically since 1972, when *Dasen* first reviewed the Piagetian cross-cultural research. Overall, population samples from non-Western cultures have been found to achieve concrete operations later, at the same time, or occasionally sooner than European and American samples. These differences in age of onset of concrete operations do not pose a threat to *Piaget's* hypothesis. The finding that was troubling 10 years ago, and that has generated a good deal of recent discussion, is the evidence that many adults in certain cultures do not attain concrete operations at all. Not surprisingly, cross-cultural research also generally has failed to find evidence of formal operational thought among non-schooled, non-Western populations.

What are Piagetians to make of this considerable variability? Interpreting the results within *Piaget's* framework, we would conclude that cognitive development is certainly not simply a matter of biological maturation. But the correctness of the other two hypotheses (equilibration or education) is difficult to determine. 'Asymptotic curves', in which development appears to have stopped for many people before achieving operational thought, do not necessarily implicate educational transmissions as a causal factor. But they do point to a greater importance of cultural factors than previously granted.

The response of Piagetian researchers to cross-cultural evidence that challenges the universality of operational thought is to make a theoretical distinction between performance on specific tasks and underlying general competence. Such a response reflects their strong belief in a general and abstract knowledge structure that underlies specific activities. *Dasen* [1977], for example, applied this competence/performance distinction to cross-cultural studies, making task performance a multiplicative outcome of underlying competence, task-specific and culture-specific knowledge. Getting at the general, abstract competence involves cutting through specific cultural knowledge and practices. A limitation of the application of the competence/performance distinction must be kept in mind: It is empirically impossible to demonstrate the *absence* of operational competence. If a child fails to demonstrate operational competence, the task can always be faulted as too difficult owing to task-specific or culture-specific knowledge that has not been attained [*Cole and Scribner*, 1974]. As a heuristic device, however, the distinction has been quite productive.

The training study has become a research strategy for assessing the validity of the competence-performance distinction (and with it Piagetian claims for the universality of competence). *Dasen* et al. [1979b], for example, tested subjects from a variety of cultures, finding that in many cases conservation was fully achieved with just a small amount of training. Younger nonconservers, however, did not show as rapid gains as older nonconservers, even though they were somewhat older than Western children who conserve. *Dasen* et al. [1979b, p. 96] offer the following framework for interpreting such studies:

> 'We can assume that, if very rapid learning is achieved through training, the "competence" or underlying operational structure must have been present but was not being expressed in the initial task performance and that the training has "actualized" the existing competence.'

Thus, training studies appear to show great promise for reconciling cross-cultural findings with *Piaget's* hypothesis.

If the results of *Dasen* et al. [1979b] could be duplicated in a large number of diverse cultures, then *Piaget's* program might be considered a success. A crucial aspect, however, would be missing from the demonstration. Little or no evidence is provided by these studies that the lags in development (relative to norms for Western children) are the consequence of an impoverishment of operatory exercise, rather than, say, lack of cultural transmissions. That is, most studies make little effort to assess the environmental conditions that co-occur with these developmental lags. Without such assessment one can only *assume* that lags result from a general impoverishment of opportunities for interacting with the environment. In other words, the developmental processes that are the topic of investigation are assumed rather than investigated.

Dissociating Environmental Factors

To measure a feature of the environment, it must first be distinguished from other features which also may affect the process of interest. Any two cultural groups differ in countless ways. Cross-cultural studies have attempted to reduce the differences by comparing two groups within a single culture that appear to differ on only one 'dimension'. But this strategy still fails to dissociate the theoretically significant factors.

For example, formal schooling has been studied extensively which is not surprising since 'educational transmission' and equilibration are the primary competing hypotheses in *Piaget's* program. *Laurendeau-Bendavid* [1977, p. 165] expressed a common view among Piagetian researchers in concluding, on the basis of studies of schooled, partly schooled, and nonschooled African children:

'In sum, school attendance appears to be a facilitating rather than a necessary condition for the attainment of concrete operations and objective causal representations, since some of the children without any schooling do attain these. On the other hand, school attendance is a necessary but not a sufficient condition for the attainment of formal operations, since only subjects with full school experience – and only a few of these – were found to have reached this level.'

These findings appear to partially support *Piaget's* hypothesis that cognitive development (at least through the concrete operational stage) is not dependent on educational transmission within classrooms. But the situation is not quite so straightforward, since educational transmission of culture-specific practices obviously goes on outside of schools. Informal education still may be a necessary condition for cognitive development.

For *Piaget's* cross-cultural program to work, the crucial factors must somehow be identified such that education (including informal education) can be distinguished from equilibration factors. But the close relation between overall level of activity and the particular cultural practices that make up that activity leads to uncertainty.

A different strategy for achieving the dissociation is illustrated by *Bovet's* [1974] study of concrete operations in rural Algeria. The importance of the study is not due to her attempt to control variables but rather to her hypotheses about the possible relations between specific everyday practices of her rural subjects and the subjects' operational development.

Bovet's [1974] method for dissociating cultural transmission processes from equilibration processes involves studying a single cultural group and observing development in the apparent absence of cultural transmission. According to her hypothesis, everyday activities are the occasion for internal 'regulatory coordinations' of the relevant concepts. Concepts that are used frequently will develop more rapidly or to a higher level. A critical part of her argument is that for this internal process to operate, the everyday activities do not, themselves, have to display the logical structure of the knowledge that develops by means of the process.

> 'It would seem that the frequent use of a variety of activities related to basic scientific concepts is beneficial for the logical development of such concepts, even when the activities are intuitive rather than logical' [*Bovet*, 1974, p. 332].

If subjects demonstrate logical operations on tests in domains in which the cultural practices do not, themselves, require logical operations, then operational development would be shown to be independent of specific cultural transmissions yet still sensitive to the opportunities for operatory exercise provided by the cultural environment.

Bovet [1974] notes that in the homes of her Algerian subjects bowls were of many different sizes and, for example, when serving food there was no attempt to assure that everyone received the same amount. She stresses that, in spite of the lack of formal measurement or concern with equivalence in their culture, rural Algerian children nevertheless do come to conserve quantity, albeit somewhat later than Genevan children. This finding suggests that children do not have to be taught the operations involved in conservation but come to them on their own through a constructive process. Adults could not have taught an operation that does not play a part in any of the practices that they transmit to their children.

While *Bovet's* argument is an important contribution to the Piagetian program, it is not entirely convincing. Unexplained is how an everyday activity can be related to a logical structure when the activity itself is not logical. Likewise, it is difficult to imagine how such knowledge could develop in abstract general form and remain entirely concealed until tapped by *Bovet's* [1974] interview procedures. Without closer scrutiny of everyday life, we cannot be confident that the practices she calls 'intuitive' do not involve 'logical' reasoning. Like the competence/performance distinction, the hypothesis that the logical basis for cultural practices will be discovered with closer scrutiny is unfalsifiable. Yet, as a heuristic assumption, it may be productive.

Bovet does argue that cognitive development is closely related to the specific practices that a culture provides. But, at the same time, she holds that the particulars of the practice are not important; the practice serves only to bring the child in contact with the materials and opportunities to interact with them. It is the child who constructs the logical system. The difficulty in holding this position can be illustrated by a study that is frequently cited in the literature as an example of the effect of familiarity on the assessment of operational skills.

Price-Williams et al. [1969] studied the effect of exposure to pottery-making on the acquisition of concrete operational thinking. They found that pottery-making experiences led to earlier development of conservation of substance, assessed with reference to transformations in the shape of a ball of clay. This early development might be attributed simply to the greater *familiarity* of the potters' children with the particular materials used. But this interpretation is challenged by a second study of children of potters in Mexico [*Steinberg and Dunn*, 1976]. No differences among children from two villages were found, even though children in one village participated in pottery-making and children in the other did not. In seeking a reason for this failure to replicate the findings of *Price-Williams* et al. [1969], *Steinberg and Dunn* [1976] call attention to the differences in the potting process in their respective populations.

In the *Price-Williams* et al. [1969] population, the production process of the potters was very similar to the classic conservation of substance task. The making of pottery by children in these villages involves fitting balls of clay into molds. The shape of the clay is transformed while the weight and the amount of clay remains constant. If problems arise, the clay is removed from the mold and returned to the original shape of a ball. Thus, transformation in form and reversibility actions hypothesized as necessary for conservation learning are practiced by this group of children. In the population studied by *Steinberg and Dunn* [1976], the production process used by the potters was to build pots by placing coils of clay one upon another, the size and number of coils varying with the pot. Thus, potting did not provide the experience of invariance.

These two studies of potters' children suggest that the kind of experience necessary for cognitive development is related to the specific concept that develops. It is not sufficient for the child simply to have opportunities to interact with the material world. Rather, it would appear to be necessary that those interactions be organized by the culture in particular ways. The use of a mold in pottery making, for example, provides for the repeated transformation of clay, illustrating the principle of reversibility. In an important sense, the concept of reversibility is entailed by the use of a mold. Such examples suggest that cognitive competence may closely model specific practices found in the culture.

The close relation between cultural practices and specific domains of cognitive competence has been demonstrated in studies by *Heron* and his colleagues [reviewed in *Dasen and Heron*, 1981], who raise questions about the 'domain consistency' of the concrete operational stage. The assessed rates of development across tasks said to measure concrete operations are not consistent across cultures. *Dasen and Heron* [1981, p. 327] conclude:

'The structure d'ensemble posited for the Genevan child does not necessarily hold elsewhere; two concepts that develop congruently in the average Genevan child may develop at very different rates in another culture, if one of them is more highly valued (i.e. is more relevant or adaptive) in that other culture'.

The cross-cultural variability in acquisition rates across subdomains has been a sufficiently robust finding to allow *Dasen* [1975] to make use of this variability to test *Berry's* [1971] eco-cultural model. *Dasen* [1975] predicted that low food-accumulating, nomadic hunting groups would develop spatial concepts more rapidly than sedentary food-accumulating populations, but that the latter would excel at conservation tasks. He reasoned that those concepts that are of functional value in a culture will have a greater chance to develop. His data from Eskimo, Australian Aborigines and an Ivory Coast agricultural population confirmed his expectations.

Dasen [1977] and *Dasen* et al. [1979a] argue that Piagetian stage theory does not necessarily imply that non-Western cultures have general deficits. While members of a culture may lag (and perhaps even reach an asymptote) in some domains, they may excel in other domains more closely related to the practices found within the culture.

The existence of relations between specific cultural practices and particular domains of cognitive development makes the cross-cultural program outlined by *Piaget* impossible to carry out. Researchers do not report overall deficits in level of interaction with the environment. Rather, they find effects related to the specific domains in which various cultures provide experience. Under these conditions, the only way to maintain a distinction between equilibration factors and factors of educational transmission would be to accept an argument such as *Bovet's* [1974] that the practices that are transmitted need not themselves make use of the logic which is expressed to the researcher in the interview. In the remainder of this paper we examine the theoretical reformulation that would be necessary if the sharp distinction between equilibration and educational transmission were modified as a solution to the problem of domain specificity in the effects of culture on cognitive development.

Domain Specificity and Piaget's Theory

The position taken by *Dasen and Heron* [1981] is quite consistent with *Piaget's* [1972] own speculations regarding the fact that a large percentage of Western individuals of normal intelligence and average social background do not function fully at the formal operational stage as measured by performance on standard formal operational tasks. *Piaget* [1972] proposed that all adults use formal operations but not in all areas at all times. Thus, in order to find evidence of formal operations, he suggests that tasks would have to be developed in areas of high interest and personal experience. Lawyers would need to be given formal operational problems in law, for example, while Polynesian navigators would be given formal operational tasks involving the relations of stars and islands. *Piaget* is optimistic that intellectual development will be universally describable in terms of his structural theory. Every culture has practices that provide experience in *some* domain, which should lead to the development of concrete and formal operations in that domain.

The Paradox of Domain Specificity

The domain-specific position represents quite a radical departure from the usual Piagetian position that regards development as change in a central psychological structure. *Dasen* [1977] points to the paradoxical nature of *Piaget's* domain-specific formulation of formal operational competence. Formal operations by their very nature are abstract and not tied to the concrete world. One would expect that such abstract knowledge would apply very generally. Yet, as *Piaget* [1972] suggests, in practice, formal operations are available only in specific domains. In fact, it is the most concrete knowledge, for example the sensorimotor conceptions of space, that has the widest application.

This paradox necessitates a recognition of two orthogonal dimensions along which knowledge can be characterized. One dimension, 'concrete to abstract', pertains to the nature of the knowledge itself, that is, the level of abstraction at which some phenomenon is understood. The other dimension, 'specific to general', pertains to the range of contexts to which the knowledge applies.

In *Piaget's* [1970] theory abstract knowledge arises from coordinations of previously uncoordinated actions or schemas. Such abstract knowledge is then more general than any of the specific (and more concrete) uncoordinated schemas. But it is apparently the case that this process of coordination operates only within specific domains that provide a sufficiently rich or concentrated array of experiences to promote or require the coordination. Within any individual's experience, only certain domains (such as those involved in the individual's occupation) would provide the necessary concentration of experience. Hence, abstractions may arise that are nevertheless domain-specific.

It is becoming recognized increasingly that an individual's knowledge is not organized as a single general structure [*Feldmann*, 1980; *Fischer* 1980; *Siegler and Richards*, 1981; *Turiel*, 1978]. When we dis-

anized general knowledge struc-
ance' distinction is no longer
pic for research, the question of
ain come to be transferred hori-
of this view, training studies like
do not tap 'underlying' compe-
fficient prompts to enable them
' to what they already know in

dence of an association between
particular domains is that units
activity. The 'domains' of a cul-
and defined within the culture.
an individual's knowledge with
ension would, to a great extent,
al activities of the culture.
distinction between equilibra-
ch is at the heart of *Piaget's* the-
ctices must be kept at a distance
mption of an indirect relation
ment is reflected in Piagetians'
ir ideas about the basic units of
Bovet, 1974] often use the term
lge that develop. An individual
pt of length' or the 'concept of
owledge appear more closely
s and logic than to domains of
h Piagetian concepts are taken
tion to the child's everyday ac-
ifferent activities may put the
h' problems, for example. All
are pooled in the development
the practical activities actually
agetians speak of domain-spe-
ge still appear to apply gener-
ice. This is so because the vari-
onto the activities themselves.
e strong influence of cultural
ation of a competence consist-

ing of practical abilities that incorporate logical principles. To maintain the distinction between equilibration and educational transmission, it is necessary to take *Bovet's* [1974] position: Cultural practices do not entail logical thinking; they simply put the child in contact with materials and other people, enabling the child to invent the logic.

A crucial task that remains for Piagetian cross-cultural research is to examine more systematically the logical operations entailed by cultural practices. *Saxe* [1982], for example, has made considerable headway in demonstrating the socio-historical basis for cognitive operations in his studies of number concepts among the Oksapmin of Papua New Guinea. Collaborating with an anthropologist, he was able to identify specific ways in which the introduction of trade stores leads to greater abstraction in the indigenous numeration system. Studies such as *Saxe's* [1982] that go beyond anecdotal accounts and that begin to utilize the techniques of cognitive anthropology in examining Piagetian concepts will provide the basis for accepting or rejecting *Bovet's* [1974] argument.

The Social Object

We have suggested that the kinds of experience that may provide 'operatory exercise' (and that can therefore be attributed to equilibration of an intra-individual or inter-individual sort) are difficult to distinguish from experiences that can be described as cultural transmission. This is so because, as the domain-specific findings suggest, operatory exercise leading to operational development always occurs in the context of culturally specific practices. This fact calls for a reassessment of *Piaget's* conception of the relation between culture and thought. Is scientific thought an inevitable natural development or is it an historically conditioned way of thinking, as many writers have suggested [*Buck-Morss,* 1975; *Greenfield,* 1976; *Luria,* 1976]? In other words, what is the relation between cognitive development that is the result of an allegedly 'natural' process of equilibration and the specific cultural practices transmitted to children?

From a theoretical perspective in sharp contrast with the Piagetian position, *El'konin* [1972] has argued that interaction with the environment in the context of learning cultural practices implies interaction with social objects rather than natural objects. In the Soviet approach, strongly influenced by *Vygotsky* [1978], an object is defined primarily in terms of its role in modes of activity in a particular culture rather than in terms of its raw physical properties. Even when children are engaged in seemingly nonsocial activity with objects, they are actually dealing with objects that are defined in a particular way by the culture into which the child is being integrated. Soviet investigators do not deny that objects can be analyzed in other ways (e.g. in terms of their role in a physical system studied in science), but they argue that these other ways of analyzing objects (that usually come somewhat later in ontogenesis) are also culturally organized (e.g. by current scientific theories). Objects are *socially defined objects* and therefore serve as a point of contact between culture and intelligence. The objects in a child's world are already transmitted by the culture, so interactions with them cannot be free of the culture's influence.

Piaget does see a close relation between individual and social action, but this relation is of a different sort than that proposed by *El'konin* [1972] (see also *Leontyev* [1981]). In *Piaget's* view, the equilibration process is always simultaneously individual and social. If we ask whether the intellectual operations are the cause or the effect of social cooperation, *Piaget* [1968] answers that it is like the question of whether the chicken appears before the egg. Social logic and individual logic constitute inseparable aspects of a single reality [*Piaget*, 1968, p. 158].

This conception of the interdependence of social and individual domains places their interaction only at the most abstract and general level. The two domains are isomorphic only when entirely free of content. *El'konin's* [1973] argument, on the other hand, is at the level of content and, therefore, implicates the cultural specifics of the socially determined function and meaning of the objects with which the child interacts. If the latter conception of social objects is accepted, it becomes all the harder to distinguish equilibration factors (whether with respect to objects, factor 2, or the social world, factor 3) from specific social factors (factor 4). The equilibration process occurs only in relation to social objects of the particular culture. Our point in this regard can be made by extending *Piaget's* [1963] biological metaphor for understanding the process of cognitive equilibration. He draws a comparison between the biological system of ingestion of food and the intellectual process of taking in cognitive experiences. The digestive system of an organism dictates which of the range of possible nutrients it can and cannot accommodate. The assimilation of acceptable nutrients will lead to slow changes in the system, which will alter the selection of future nutrients. Similarly, the intellectual system dictates which of a range of possible intellectual experiences it can and cannot assimilate. The assimilation of acceptable experiences will lead to slow changes in the system, altering future ability to assimilate.

The availability of biological nourishment and intellectual experience, however, are not determined solely by the efforts of individuals. Foods that are made available to children are carefully selected, processed and prepared for children by their parents and by their culture. Just as parents carefully prepare food for children, so, too, parents (and others in the child's environment) prepare and constrain the type of intellectual experiences to which the child will be exposed. By analogy to the prepared baby-food or food-processing devices available to parents, the social distribution of knowledge in any society provides normative guides for the preparation and distribution of 'baby experiences' that will lead to the intellectual growth valued by the culture. It is in these ways and in terms of these cultural practices that all reality can be said to be a social reality.

If logical principles are contained in the particular practices children learn as they grow, does this necessarily eliminate a constructive process such as equilibration? *Piaget* [1970, p. 715] is particularly concerned that children be allowed to discover things on their own.

> 'Remember also that each time one prematurely teaches a child something he could have discovered for himself, that child is kept from inventing it and consequently from understanding it completely. This obviously does not mean the teacher should not devise experimental situations to facilitate the pupil's invention.'

If some practice provides operatory exercise, then learning the practice in the first place would be an occasion for discovering the principles on which the practice is based. While the principles would not have to be explicitly taught, the practice would be an occasion for learning, somewhat in the same way that teachers or experimenters can set up situations designed to provide the right kind of practice. Here again, the Vygotskian approach provides a useful formulation of such a phenomenon.

Vygotsky [1978] argues that development follows learning, rather than the other way around as *Piaget* would have it. Learning specific cultural practices under the guidance and with the support of others provides the occasion for children to have the experiences necessary for the more fundamental and permanent kind of development change *Piaget* is concerned with. It may well be the case, as *Piaget* [1970] argues, that children cannot learn things on their own for which they are not developmentally prepared. But with adult help children can be involved in activities they could not engage in on their own. The question can be asked: How are occasions organized such that children who are preoperational, for example, can nevertheless participate in social occasions requiring conservation? If a nonconserver were to be sharing the food in a home in which equal distribution among siblings were practiced, then any wrong assumptions he or she may have about what is the same amount would be quickly pointed out. Or the child would be given 'help' by parents or older siblings, such that the portions would be shared equally. In such a case, conservation of quantity is presupposed by the adult or older child in the way sharing is accomplished and in the way the younger child is brought into the activity. Conservation becomes part of the interaction [*Griffin* el al., 1981]. And these interactions need not be at all coercive. The adult and child are simply cooperating to accomplish the activity.

Vygotsky's [1978] theory emphasizes the socio-historical context of the acquisition of knowledge. In this respect, his theory appears opposed to *Piaget's* constructivist theory, which emphasizes individual invention through equilibration. The two theories of knowledge acquisition can coexist, however, if it is supposed that the logical basis for cultural practices is not explicitly taught but constructed by the child in the course of learning to play a gradually larger role in the practice. In this sense, children's active contribution to their own development through equilibration may still be distinguishable from overt attempts to transmit knowledge through instruction. Opportunities for equilibration occur within specific contexts and these contexts have been organized by social and cultural forces to influence the course of development. This formulation of the relation between cultural practices and equilibration raises questions about the universality of operational development, which has been a central feature of *Piaget's* theory. Establishing that there are universals in the development of human thought will require more thorough examination of the context-embedded process as well as the products of cognitive development.

Our review of Piagetian cross-cultural research has pointed to the evidence that operational development is closely tied to the cultural practices to which the developing child is exposed. This fact suggests that the child's learning of these practices under the guidance of others provides the context of development. Cultural transmission, then, is not a separate process in addition to a process such as equilibration but rather supplies the raw materials on which the latter operates. Further study of cultural practices and their transmission may therefore shed light on fundamental questions concerning the process of cognitive development.

Summary

In this chapter we examine the implications of recent cross-cultural research for *Piaget's* theory and its underlying assumptions about the relation between cognition and culture. *Piaget* proposed to gather cross-cultural evidence in order to test his hypothesis that a universal equilibration process accounts for cognitive development. *Piaget's* attempt to dissociate specific educational transmission from the equilibration process necessitates that cultures vary in overall amount of opportunity to interact with the environment, considered by *Piaget* as the major factor governing the rate at which the equilibration process occurs. Cross-cultural researchers, however, have found considerable variability related to specific cultural practices but have been unable to identify differences in overall amount of interaction. While the outcome of the research program is, so far, inconclusive, the finding of specific rather than general differences between cultures leads to a paradox for *Piaget's* initial formulation. If knowledge acquisition is domain-specific rather than general, as the research evidence has suggested, and cultural variation is specific rather than general, then it is difficult if not impossible to distinguish specific education from the more general equilibration process. The resolution we propose is based on *Vygotsky's* socio-historical theory in which cognitive development arises out of specific social-cultural experiences. These experiences provide the raw materials on which a process such as equilibration may operate. We argue for greater attention in cross-cultural research to the logical structure inherent in the cultural practices themselves.

Acknowledgements

Preparation of this chapter was supported by grants from the Carnegie Corporation and the Ford Foundation (780-0639A) to *Michael Cole*. We are grateful to *Michael Cole* for constructing in many ways a 'zone of proximal development' without which we could not have gotten through the task of writing this paper. We are grateful as well to *Marsha DeForest*, who contributed to an earlier version of this paper and to *Andrea Petitto*, who provided us with background research. *Bud Mehan, Marsha DeForest* and *Andrea Petitto* provided useful comments on earlier versions.

References

Berry, J.W: Ecological and spacial factors in spacial perceptual development. Can. J. behav. Sci. *3:* 324-336 (1971).
Bovet, M.C.: Cognitive processes among illiterate children and adults; in Berry, Dasen, Culture and cognition: readings in cross-cultural studies, pp. 311-334 (Methuen, London 1974).
Buck-Morss, S.: Socio-economic bias in Piaget's theory and its implications for cross-cultural studies. Hum. Dev. *18:* 35-49 (1975).
Cole, M.; Scribner, S.: Culture and thought: a psychological introduction (Wiley, New York 1974).
Dasen, P.R.: Cross-cultural Piagetian research: a summary. J. cross-cultural Psychol. *3:* 29-39 (1972).
Dasen, P.R.: Concrete operational development in three cultures. J. cross-cultural Psychol. *6:* 156-172 (1975).
Dasen, P.R.: Cross-cultural cognitive development: the cultural aspects of Piaget's theory. Ann. N.Y. Acad. Sci. *285* 332-337 (1977).
Dasen, P.R.; Berry, J.W.; Witkin, H.A.: The use of developmental theories cross-culturally; in Eckensberger, Lonner, Poortinga, Cross-cultural contributions to psychology, pp. 69-82 (Swets Publishing, Amsterdam 1979a).
Dasen, P.R.; Heron, A.: Cross-cultural tests of Piaget's theory; in Triandis, Heron, Handbook of cross-cultural psychology: developmental psychology, vol. 14, pp. 295-342 (Allyn & Bacon, Boston 1981).
Dasen, P.R.; Ngini, L.; Laballee, M.: Cross-cultural training studies of concrete operations; in Eckensberger, Lonner, Poortinga, Cross-cultural contributions to psychology, pp. 94-104 (Swets & Zeitlinger, Amsterdam 1979b).
El'konin, D.B.: Toward the problem of stages in the mental development of the child. Soviet Psychol. *10:* 225-251 (1972).
Feldmann, D.H.: Beyond universals in cognitive development (Ablex, Norwood 1980).
Fischer, K.W.: A theory of cognitive development: The control and construction of hierarchies of skills. Psychol. Rev. *87:* 477-531 (1980).
Greenfield, P.M.: On culture and conservation; in Bruner, Oliver, Greenfield, Studies in cognitive growth, pp. 225-256 (Wiley, New York 1966).
Greenfield, P.M.: Cross-cultural research and Piagetian theory: paradox and progress; in Riegel, Meacham, The developing individual in a changing world: historical and cultural issues, vol. 1, pp. 322-333 (Aldine, Chicago 1976).
Griffin, P.; Newman, D.; Cole, M.: Activities, actions and formal operations: a Vygotskian analysis of a Piagetian task. Proc. Meet. of the Int. Soc. for the Study of Behavioral Development, Toronto 1981.
Laurendeau-Bendavid, M: Culture, schooling and cognitive development: a comparative study of children in French Canada and Rwanda; in Dasen, Piagetian psychology: cross-cultural contributions (Gardner Press, New York 1977).
Leontyev, A.N.: Problems of the development of the mind (Progress Publishers, Moscow 1981).
Luria, A.R.: Cognitive development (Harvard University Press, Cambridge 1976).

Mosheni, N.: La comparaison des réactions aux épreuves d'intelligence en Iran et en Europe; unpublished thesis, (1966).
Piaget, J.: The origins of intelligence in children (Norton, New York 1963).
Piaget, J.: Six psychological studies (Vintage, New York 1968).
Piaget, J.: Piaget's theory; in Mussen, Carmichael's manual of child psychology; 3rd ed. (Wiley, New York 1970).
Piaget, J.: Intellectual evolution from adolescence to adulthood. Hum. Dev. *15:* 1–12 (1972).
Piaget, J.: To understand is to invent (Grossman, New York 1973).
Piaget, J.: Need and significance of cross-cultural studies in genetic psychology; in Berry, Dasen, Culture and cognition: readings in cross-cultural psychology, pp. 299-310 (Methuen, London 1974).
Price-Williams, D.; Gordon, W.; Ramírez, M.: Skill and conservation: a study of pottery-making children. Devl.Psychol. *1:* 769 (1969).
Saxe, G.B.: Culture and the development of numerical cognition: studies among the Oksapmin of Papua New Guinea; in Brainerd, Children's logical and mathematical cognition (Springer, New York, in press, 1982).
Siegler, R.S.; Richards, D.D.: The development of intelligence; in Sternberg, Handbook of human intelligence (Cambridge University Press, Cambridge 1981).
Steinberg, B.M.; Dunn, L.A.: Conservation competence and performance in Chiapas. Hum. Dev. *19:* 14-25 (1976).
Turiel, E.: The development of concepts of social structure; in Glick, Clarke-Stewart, The development of social understanding, pp. 25-108 (Gardner, New York 1978).
Vygotsky, L.S.: Mind in society: the development of higher psychological processes (Harvard University Press, Cambridge 1978).

Author Index

Achenbach, T.M. 7, 11, 12, 21
Achinstein, P. 14, 18
Anderson, J.R. 61, 72, 128
Aries, P. VIII, 44
Arnold, W.J. 1
Ausubel, D.P. 21

Baer, D.M. 6
Baldwin, A.L. 7, 12, 17
Baldwin, J.M. 54, 102, 107
Baltes, P. 7, 11, 14, 17, 18, 21, 22
Becker, E. 48
Bell, D. 46–48
Berger, P.L. 32
Bergmann, G. 11, 22
Bergson, H. 55, 67
Bernard, J. 45
Bernstein, M. 114
Berry, J.W. 140, 145
Bertalanffy, L. von 57
Bevan, W. 48
Bijou, S.W. 6
Birren, J.W. 10, 11, 22, 128
Bisanz, J. 69, 71, 72, 74
Bischof, N. 56, 61
Blumenthal, A.L. 55
Boli-Bennett, J. 47
Bossom, J. 66
Botwinick, J. 125

Bovet, M.C. 142–148
Bowlby, J. 61
Brainerd, C.J. 12, 13, 21, 22, 84
Braithwaite, R. 13
Branca, P. 45
Bromley, D.B. 11, 17, 22
Bronfenbrenner, U. 10
Bronowski, J. 116
Broughton, J.M. 35, 111
Brown, A.L. 97, 99, 112, 115
Brown, H. 2
Bruner, J.S. 70, 71
Buck-Morss, S. 33, 148
Burt, R.A. 47
Buss, A.R. 34
Byrne, D.F. 64

Campbell, D.T. 13
Carnap, R. 11
Case, R. XI, 69–71, 74, 83, 89–98, 103–105, 108
Cattell, P.B. 7
Chandler, M.J. 125
Charles, D.C. VII
Chestnut, R. 84
Christie, A. 123
Clayton, V. 118, 128
Cole, M. 140, 151
Conway, B.E. 114

Cook, J. 124
Cornelius, S.W. 17, 18, 21
Cronbach, L.J. 14, 33, 48

Danto, A. 23
Darrow, C.M. 118, 119
Dasen, P.R. 135, 139–141, 144–147
Degler, C. 45
DeLoache, J. 97
Dennett, D. 104
Denny-Brown, D. 65
Donzelot, J. 47, 48
Draguns, S. 66
Dray, W. 22
Dunn, L.A. 143, 144

Edelstein, W. 48
Elder, G.H., Jr. VIII, 33
Elkind, D. 125
El'konin, D.B. 148, 149
Emler, N.P. 34
Eriksen, C.W. 14
Erikson, E.H. 118

Feigl, H. 11
Feldmann, D.H. 146
Feyerabend, P.K. 9
Fischer, D.H. 44
Fischer, K.W. 57
Fishbein, H.D. 76

Author Index

Fiske, D.W. 13
Fitzgerald, J.M. 120, 122
Flavell, J.H. 60, 66, 73, 84, 97, 98
Fokkema, S. 75
Fremont, J. 124
Furth, H.G. 37, 131

Gadlin, H. VIII, 45
Gagné, R.M. 68
Gallie, W.B. 23
Garner, W.R. 14
Geiss, M.F. 54
Gelman, R. 84
Gentner, D. 58
Gergen, K.J. I, III, IX
Gesell, A. 83
Getzels, J.W. 128
Gewirtz, J.L. 7, 11, 17, 21
Gilligan, C. 118
Gillis, J.R. 44
Glaser, R. 75
Glick, P.C. 44
Gordon, W. 143, 144
Greenfield, P.M. 136, 148
Greeno, J.G. 72
Greven, P. 44
Grief, E.B. 60
Griffin, P. 151
Grinder, R. 54
Gutting, G. 1, 2

Habermas, J. 31, 38–40, 50, 111
Hake, H.W. 14
Halford, G.S. 70
Hall, G.S. 32, 83
Hanson, N.R. 8, 18, 23
Harre, R. 14
Hayes, J.R. 72, 73
Hayes-Roth, B. 72
Heelan, P.A. 2
Held, D. 32, 42, 43
Held, R. 66
Hempel, C.G. 10, 11, 14–16, 18, 20, 22
Heron, A. 135, 144

Hesse, M. 14
Hilts, P.J. 116
Hogan, R.T. 34
Horn, J.L. 122
Hull, C.L. 16, 21, 56

Iannotti, R.J. 127
Inhelder, B. 69, 94
Ives, S.W. 21

Jackson, J.H. 56, 71
Jenkins, J.J. 112
Jerison, H.J. 56

Kahneman, D. 71
Kail, R. 57, 69, 71, 72, 74
Kaplan, A. 14, 18, 22
Kaplan, B. 59, 60, 64, 65
Keat, R. 38, 39, 43
Kendler, H.H. 1, 5, 9
Kessen, W. VIII, 33, 47, 48, 85
Ketron, J.L. 114
Kett, J. VIII, 44
Kimble, G. 5
Kirasic, K.C. 57
Kisiel, T.J. 2
Kitchener, R.F. 3, 4, 6, 19, 21, 22, 25, 37, 39, 72
Klahr, D. 61, 63, 69, 71–74, 89, 90
Klein, E.B. 118, 119
Koch, S. 1, 11, 21
Kockelmans, J.J. 2
Kohlberg, L. 35, 60
Kovach, J.K. 53
Kuhn, D. 96
Kuhn, T. 1, 8, 19, 32
Kurtines, W. 60

Labouvie-Vief, G. 118
Lakatos, I. 18
Lasch, C. 47, 48
Lashley, K.S. 123
Laurendeau-Bendavid, M. 141
Lawler, R.W. 74

Lefkowitz, M.R. 129
Leontyev, A.N. 149
Lerner, R.M. 7, 9, 11, 12, 17, 18, 22, 70, 72
Lesgold, A.M. 75
Levinson, D.J. 118, 119
Levinson, M.H. 118, 119
Lewin, K. 82
Liebert, D.E. 115
Liebert, R.M. 115
Lipsitt, L.P. 21
Looft, W.R. 10, 115
Lorenz, K.Z. 65
Luckman, T. 32
Lull, R. 115
Luria, A.R. 67, 148

McArthur, C.C. 118, 119
McCandless, B.R. 7, 11, 17, 22, 54
McCarthy, J. 47
McCarthy, T. 38, 40
MacCorquodale, K. 13
McKee, B. 118, 119
MacLean, P.D. 57
Mackworth, N.H. 128
McMullin, E. 19
Mandelbaum, M. 22
Mandler, G. 67
Marshall, J.F. 72
Martin, W. 84
Marx, M. 7
Meacham, J.A. III, 117, 119, 127, 131
Meehl, P.E. 13, 14
Merton, R.K. 32
Meyer, J.W. 47
Miller, J.G. 65, 66
Milner, E. 57, 67
Moessinger, P. 130
Montagu, A. 116
Mosheni, N. 138
Murphy, G. 53
Murphy, J.M. 118
Mussen, P.H. 10

Neches, R. 72, 73

Author Index

Nesselroade, J.R. 7, 11, 14, 17, 18, 21, 22
Newell, A. 61
Newman, D. 151
Nickels, T. 25
Novikoff, A.B. 56

Oppenheimer, R. 66
Overton, W.F. 7, 11, 17, 22, 55, 56, 61

Pap, A. 14
Parke, R. 44
Pascual-Leone, J. 70, 74, 89-93, 103
Pattee, J. 57
Pellegrino, J.W. 75
Pepper, S.C. 112
Perry, W.G. 118
Phelps, E. 96
Piaget, J. XI, 12, 25, 31, 35-43, 50, 54, 56-59, 63, 65, 69, 70, 75, 81, 83-94, 99-108, 115, 118, 129, 131, 135-142, 145-150, 152
Plato 127
Platt, A. 47
Popper, K. 7, 8
Price-Williams, D. 143, 144

Rabbitt, P.M.A. 72
Radnitzsky, G. 2
Ramirez, M. 143, 144
Rappoport, L. 18
Reder, L.M. 128
Reese, H.W. 7, 11, 14, 17, 18, 21, 22, 61
Reichenbach, H. 3
Reinert, G.P. VII
Renner, V.J. II
Resnick, L.B. 70, 75
Ribot, R. 55
Richards, D.D. 146
Riegel, K.F. VIII, 32, 55, 111, 112, 115, 129
Riesman, D. 46

Rombach, H. 2
Rosenthal, B.G. 113, 114
Rosinski, R.R. 66
Rozin, P. 57

Saari, D.G. 71
Samelson, F. 112
Sameroff, A.J. 33
Sampson, E.E. 33-37, 119
Saxe, G.B. 148
Scandura, J. 98
Schneewind, K.A. 2
Scribner, S. 140
Scriven, M. 23
Sears, R. VII, 31, 48, 107
Sechenov, I.M. 65
Seiffert, H. 2
Selman, R.L. 64
Senn, M.J.E. VII, 31, 48, 85
Sennett, R. 45
Seyffarth, H. 65
Siegel, A.W. 55, 57, 60, 61, 67, 68, 73
Siegler, R.S. 63, 70, 73, 89, 106, 115, 146
Simon, H.A. 58, 61, 68
Skinner, B.F. 6, 20
Skinner, E.A. 17, 18
Skolnick, A. 47
Slobodkin, L.B. 66
Smith, E.E. 56
Socrates 126-128
Sorell, G.T. 17, 18
Spence, J.T. 5
Spence, K.W. 5, 9, 21
Spencer, H. X, 54, 55, 56, 59, 64, 75
Spiker, C.C. 7, 11, 17, 22, 60
Steinberg, B.M. 143, 144
Steiner, G.Y. 32, 47
Sternberg, R. 98, 114
Stevens, S.S. 11
Stone, L. 44
Sullivan, E.V. 21, 34
Suppe, F. 16, 18
Sutherland, T.W. 56

Teitelbaum, P. 65, 72
Thomas, R.M. 7
Tolman, E.C. 13, 21
Toulmin, S. 18, 25
Turiel, E. 146
Turner, M. 1
Tweney, R.D. 25
Twitchell, T.E. 65, 66
Tyack, D.B. 45

Vaillant, G.E. 118, 119
Van den Berg, A. 43
Vygotsky, L.S. XII, 148, 150-152

Waddington, C.H. 69
Wallace, S. 61, 63, 71, 74, 89, 90
Weimer, W.B. 1
Weiss, P.A. 61
Werner, H. 54, 55, 59, 60, 64, 66, 73, 75
White, S.H. 54, 60, 61, 67, 68, 73, 82, 91, 106
Wilford, J.N. 124
Wilkinson, A. 63
Willis, S.L. 14, 17, 21
Wilson, W.H. 70
Witkin, H.A. 140, 141, 145, 147
Wohlwill, J.F. 60, 70
Wolman, B. 1
Woodward, J. 22
Wozniak, R. 102

Yates, F.A. 115
Youniss, J. 37, 39, 119

Subject Index

Adulthood 125
Advertising 84
Attentional capacity 71

Behaviorism 6, 9, 21, 83
Biological factors 136

Causal explanation 104
Cautiousness 126
Cognition 25, 35, 81–108, 111–132, 135–152
Concrete operations 64, 70, 82, 95, 144
Constructivism 99–103, 108
Contextualism 4
Critical theory 31–52
Cross-cultural comparison 135–152
Cultural practices 137, 146
Curiosity 125, 130

Deductive-nomological model 20
Developmental analysis 53–75
Differentiation 56, 59, 64, 73
Domain specificity 145

Educational transmission 137
Empiricism 1, 6, 14, 38
Equilibration 40, 69, 93, 105, 129, 132, 142
Explanation 12, 53–75, 86, 104

Formal operations 36, 115, 146

Generalizability 31, 50

Hermeneutics 38
Hierarchical organization 56–58
Historical context 113
History of science 1–26
Hypotheses 7
Hypothetical constructs 13

Individualism 34, 35, 43
Induction 5
Information processing 62, 68, 71, 81, 89–91
Integration 56–58, 73
Intelligence 112–119
Invariant sequence 58

Knowledge 38, 111–132

Learning theory 83
Life cycle 45

Memory 56
Metacognition 97
Methodological behaviorism 9, 10, 21
M-power 70, 93–96

Old age 126
Operationism 10

Perception 66

Subject Index

Philosophy of science 1-26, 33
Positivism 1-26, 34
Praxis 4, 34
Prediction 8

Reflexes 65
Rigidity 126

School attendance 137
Scientific method 1-26
Scientism 36
Self-regulation 39, 42, 68, 81-108
Sequence analysis 63-68
Social construction 50
Social context 43, 113, 148-151

Social history 43-49, 137
Social transactions 39, 130-131
Socialization 137, 148-151
Sociocultural factors 148-151
Sociology 34, 47, 50
Stages 12, 53-75, 85-88, 101
Strategies 95-97
Structure-function analysis 61
Systems 56

Task analysis 70, 92
Time 60
Transition 68-71

Wisdom 111

LIBRARY OF DAVIDSON COLLEGE